Overcoming the trauma of betrayal, helping my partner recover from sex addiction, and mending our relationship

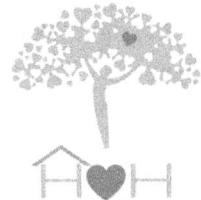

We struggled to grasp the effects that sexual addiction had on both our marriage and my health when we first visited Dr. Fai at House of Hope. At first, I had no idea what sex addiction was or why my spouse had betrayed me over such a prolonged period of time, and in secret. While desperately attempting to save our marriage, my spouse was in a state of denial and shame. We were both devastated and at a crossroads. I didn't understand why I felt the way I did or acted the way I did. I was torn between staying and leaving. The word "why" was the centre of all of my questions. Dr Fai made a brief phone call to us before meeting us in person and asked to talk with my husband and I separately. I felt straight away that we would be in good hands thanks to her soothing words and knowledge. By explaining that I was displaying trauma responses, she normalised my feelings, pain and agonising suffering. Although honest, she was empathetic and exactly what we needed. She scheduled a longer face-to-face appointment with us after the phone interview. Although I was anxious, I was eager to know the answers. On the other hand, my spouse was attempting to sabotage the appointment by coming up with excuses. He later admitted to me that after speaking with Dr. Fai on the phone, he realised it was she who would stop him from lying or manipulating his way out of recovery which scared him.

Although daunting, our first intensive session was also full with solutions and optimism for the both of us and our relationship. I thought I had finally found someone who could help me get past my pain and loss. I no longer felt alone. My husband was introduced to a secure community and given clear instructions regarding sobriety. A few short months later, we have both changed, and we are forging a new relationship. We have access to resources and tools, and we know how to deal with daily triggers and uncertainty. Both my husband and I are now more educated about sex addiction, its root causes and impacts. Considering daily challenges caused by this vicious disease, every session brings us closer together and give us more healing. I firmly believe that our children would have divorced parents if it weren't for Dr. Fai. Instead, I'm motivated and decided to stay, knowing that I won't regret it. My husband is not perfect, but he is progressing, we are not perfect but we are growing together and improving. Many thanks, Dr. Fai

Veronica and Marc

THE PAIN AND BETRAYAL TRAUMA CAUSED BY SEXUAL ADDICTION

An Unwanted Gift That Keeps Giving

Dr Fai Seyed Aghamiri

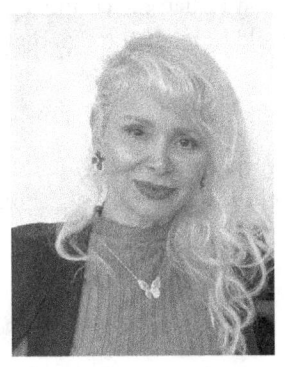

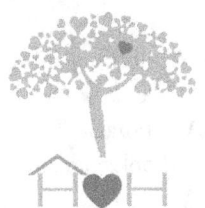

First published by Ultimate World Publishing 2023
Copyright © 2023 Dr. Fai Seyed Aghamiri

ISBN

Paperback: 978-1-922982-03-2
Ebook: 978-1-922982-04-9

Dr. Fai Seyed Aghamiri has asserted her rights under the Copyright, Designs and Patents Act 1988 to be identified as the author of this work. The information in this book is based on the author's experiences and opinions. The publisher specifically disclaims responsibility for any adverse consequences which may result from use of the information contained herein. Permission to use information has been sought by the author. Any breaches will be rectified in further editions of the book.

All rights reserved. No part of this publication may be reproduced, stored in or introduced into a retrieval system, or transmitted in any form, or by any means (electronic, mechanical, photocopying, recording or otherwise) without the prior written permission of the author. Any person who does any unauthorised act in relation to this publication may be liable to criminal prosecution and civil claims for damages. Enquiries should be made through the publisher.

Cover design: Ultimate World Publishing
Layout and typesetting: Ultimate World Publishing
Editor: Vanessa McKay
Cover image: Sergey Nivens-Shutterstock.com

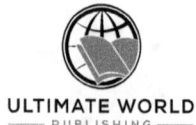

Ultimate World Publishing
Diamond Creek,
Victoria Australia 3089
www.writeabook.com.au

Dedication

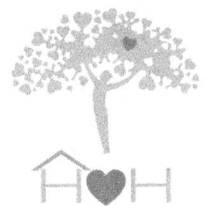

This book is dedicated to my Heavenly Father, Jesus, my saviour, who gave me the courage and zeal to serve Him by providing a platform for the betrayed partners to be heard. My life's trajectory was altered by learning about my one true God. Therefore, I commit all my work, devotion, praying, and serving in His honour.

I also dedicate my book to all the betrayed partners who valiantly continue on this challenging path, showing me and everyone else that they matter and are capable.

'Leave your troubles with the Lord, and he will defend you; he never lets honest people be defeated.'

(Psalm 55:22)

Contents

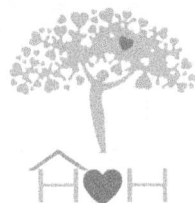

Dedication	v
Introduction	ix
CHAPTER 1: Sex addiction spectrum, risk factors and presenting signs	1
CHAPTER 2: Living with a sex addict	21
CHAPTER 3: Your sex addict partner's intimacy dysfunction	47
CHAPTER 4: Discovery & Disclosure	53
CHAPTER 5: Betrayal trauma caused by discovery and disclosure of sex addiction	59
CHAPTER 6: The multifaceted effects of betrayal trauma	69
CHAPTER 7: Betrayal trauma shatters	87
CHAPTER 8: What are triggers and when will they stop?	95
CHAPTER 9: Why polygraph?	101
CHAPTER 10: Grief and loss induced by betrayal trauma	113
CHAPTER 11: Should you stay or should you go?	129
CHAPTER 12: What are boundaries	133
CHAPTER 13: Holistic treatment plan based on betrayal trauma model	147

References	161
About Author	167
Services and Offers	169
Peer reviewed Publications	170
Other books by Dr Fai Seyed	171

Introduction

While neither role is gender exclusive, for the sake of simplicity I have used feminine pronouns for the betrayed partner and masculine pronouns for the sex addict.

When you find out about your partner's infidelity or sex addiction, you can experience a tidal wave of intense emotions. Betrayed partners often struggle for a long time to regain control over the unstable emotions brought on by unwanted thoughts, triggers, and reminders long after the initial shock and confusion of discovery or disclosure of such behaviours. I frequently witness the agonising pain and despair of the betrayed partners. These people have experienced a particular type of trauma known as betrayed trauma brought on by sex addiction. It can be so profoundly soul crushing that it alters a person's experience in ways that go beyond what can be recovered. It is essential for recovery to comprehend how and why the experience of sex addiction linked infidelity impacts our brain and behaviour and how this trauma can result in dysfunctional relational patterns and a variety of negative consequences for the wounded partner.

Trauma from betrayal causes Post Traumatic Stress Disorder (PTSD) symptoms: intrusive thoughts, avoidance, and hyperarousal are some symptoms of betrayal trauma. Intrusive thoughts are persistent and unwelcomed upsetting memories of the traumatic event and include nightmares and flashbacks, in which the horrific occurrence is relived as if it is happening again. Avoidance can take the form of attempting to stop thinking or talking about the traumatic experience as well as avoiding places, activities, or other people who remind them of the trauma. Chronic jitteriness, being always on high alert for danger, trouble falling asleep, being easily startled, having trouble focusing, and being irritable are just a few of the signs of hyperarousal.

Trauma from betrayal can literally alter the physiology due to the neurobiological changes that take place in the limbic system, which affect mood and behaviour. These alterations lead the body to enter a response of fight, flight, freeze or occasionally collapse. The brain may continue to receive reminders for a long time after the initial discovery or disclosure, flooding it with adrenaline and cortisol. This is one of the reasons why the trauma brain finds it so difficult to process the traumatic incident and afterwards refuses to relax its vigilance. As a result, The PTSD symptoms are brought on and maintained by this intensified sense of anxiety and grief. The discovery or disclosure of a partner's sex addiction frequently results in betrayed partners suffering from emotional, physical, sexual, spiritual, and relational (social) repercussions.

Introduction

Furthermore, because trauma linked grief is so complex and multidimensional, it requires a long time of intentional recovery. Betrayed trauma can induce trauma responses such as:

- Grief and loss.
- Detective mindset.
- Feeling like a fool.
- Emotional instability.
- Endless triggers.
- Isolation, shame and social embarrassment.
- Invalidation at church and faith based communities, a push to immaturely forgive.
- Lack of boundaries and accountabilities.
- Lack of self-trust and trusting others.
- Unhealthy behaviours and habits.
- Hysterical hypersexuality and trauma bonding.
- Wanting to connect while dreading connection.
- Uncertainty of staying or exiting the relationship.
- Inability to dream about the future.

Finally, betrayed partners frequently exhibit rage, sadness, anxiety, and emotional instability, and are often characterized by society as neurotic, crazy and irrational. But all of these behaviours, are responses to trauma. She is not crazy, she has been TRAUMATIZED.

CHAPTER 1

Sex addiction spectrum, risk factors and presenting signs

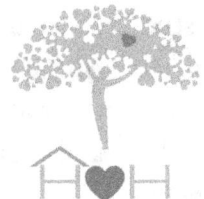

Sex addiction was first recognised for clinical purposes in the 1980s, and patient numbers have rapidly increased in recent years. According to studies, sex addiction affects somewhere between three to six percent of people, with men making up a disproportionately large share of those affected (approximately 80%). The fact that there are currently no official statistics available on the precise prevalence of sex addiction in Australia is important to note. The sole researcher to date who has examined this phenomena and its effects on the lived experiences and wellbeing of female partners is the author of this book.

Addiction is characterised as a main, persistent brain disorder that stimulates the reward, motivation, and memory-related circuitry. This definition has been provided by the American Society of Addiction Medicine to encompass both substances and behaviours. The term "addiction" is frequently used to refer to problem behaviours such as pathological gambling, computer addiction, pathological preoccupation with video games, and uncontrolled use of substances like drugs or alcohol, eating disorders and sexual addictions.

Someone who pathologically seeks pleasure and/or relief through substance use or other behaviours, such as sexual compulsivity, has a malfunctioning reward system in their brain. Some individuals who engage in behaviours that may affect their brains' reward circuitry also experience a lack of control and other indicators of addiction. According to studies, sexual and drug addiction are caused by the same brain mechanisms. In other words, compulsive sexual behaviours and heroin both have the same impact on the brain. Alcoholics, heroin addicts, and sex addicts all experience the same dopamine drunkenness.

The term "sex addiction" is used to describe compulsive sexual behaviour, porn addiction, compulsive sexual behaviour disorder, or hypersexuality.

Sex addiction is a spectrum, and while different sex addicts may appear with different symptoms, they all have a number of things in common. Sex addicts engage in a variety of sexual behaviours, masturbation and excessive use of pornography. Because there are various variations in presentation, it could seem challenging to characterise sex addiction. But it's vital to understand that SA (sexual addiction) is a blanket term for all compulsive sexual behaviours.

Sex addiction spectrum, risk factors and presenting signs

The compulsive component encompasses a variety of sexual pleasure-seeking behaviours. The cognitive-emotional aspect of sexual addiction includes sexual obsession, guilt feelings, the desire to block out unpleasant thoughts, loneliness, low self-esteem, shame, secrecy about sexual activity, justifications for continuing to engage in sexual activity, an inability to stop, and a lack of control over a number of aspects of their life.

- Sex addiction is a term used to describe a wide range of behaviours, including but not limited to:
- Compulsive masturbation.
- Compulsive porn consumption.
- Multiple affairs, sexual partners, and one night stands.
- Engaging in risky and unsafe sex.
- Cybersex.
- Meeting with sex workers.
- Sexting.
- Bestiality (performing sexual acts with animals).
- Using chat lines, dating websites, and social media to interact with people with sexual intent.
- Flirting.
- Visiting massage parlours or strip clubs.
- Using hidden cameras to record and spy on people while they engage in sexual activities without either their knowledge or consent.
- Watching individuals get dressed.

Main categories of sex addiction:

Anonymous sex: being attracted to someone merely because they are a stranger and treating them like a conquest rather than a real lover.

Fantasy sex: putting too much time and effort into fantasising about having sex, especially with a perfect partner. These powerful imaginations frequently prevent the sex addict from experiencing any type of intimacy with a partner.

Paid sex: enables a sexual addict to have nearly endless sexual partners. Sexual addicts are drawn to both the potential for ongoing sexual stimulation and the thrill of engaging in covert or risky conduct. Another type of paid sex is engaging in phone sex.

Voyeurism: spying on those who are not expecting it. Going to peep shows or watching pornographic media are also examples of the popular sex addiction known as voyeurism.

Intrusive sex: uninvited sexually suggestive physical contact, such as rubbing up against someone.

Exploitive sex: sexual contact with those who are more vulnerable, such as children or the disabled. Being able to control the victim gives the sex addict satisfaction.

Seductive sex: acting as if they are conquering someone else. For those who engage in seductive sex, getting others to engage in sex with them is satisfying. The addict could have multiple relationships going on at once and is dependent on the rush of pursuit and triumph.

Exhibitionism: displaying one's privates and taking pleasure in the reactions of others. Participating in a peep show or exposing oneself in a bar may fall under this category. Because there is always a chance of getting caught, this is a dangerous sort of sex addiction.

Trade sex: providing sex to others in exchange for money, goods, or narcotics. Because they can demand money for sex from others, sex addicts might feel powerful and in control.

Compulsive sexual behaviour or sex addiction can have terrible repercussions and cause great emotional suffering. Some people may ask if there is such a thing as a sex addiction? The response is YES! Compulsive sexual conduct is a difficult reality for many people who live with it and it extends beyond mere desire. Numerous researchers have looked into the causes of sex addiction and how background elements like gender and personality type can influence how sex addiction develops. Despite efforts to avoid these recurring sexual cravings and behaviours, they are among the signs of this brain disease which cause tremendous mental suffering and eventually impact a person's physical and mental health.

Risk factors:

A number of ideas explain the risk factors for sex addiction. One of these is attachment theory, which claims that persons with anxious or avoidant attachment utilise fantasy or sexual addiction as a substitute for intimacy because they are fearful of it.

The opportunity, attachment, and trauma model (Hall, 2013) builds upon the attachment model by adding four additional elements: opportunity, attachment, trauma, and a combination of attachment and trauma. The availability and accessibility of sexual activities or triggers, such as pornography and online sex, may increase the desire to partake in sexual pleasure in people with sex addiction. Second, early attachment trauma or injury, particularly with a cross-gender parent, is the basis of sex addiction. Third, trauma can lead to the development of sex addiction, whether or not an attachment injury has already occurred. Last but not least, sex addiction is influenced by biological, emotional, religious, social, and cultural factors. Most notably, research has shown that viewing pornography is associated with impulsivity and compulsivity, as well as the emergence of sex addiction in both men and women.

Additional risk factors for the emergence of sex addiction include:

- Co-occurring or primary mental health issues (such as depression, ADHD, dyslexia, border line personality disorder, autism or bipolar disorder).
- Dysfunctional family system.
- Brain's chemical imbalances.
- Abuse (emotional, physical or sexual abuse).
- Past experience of abandonment.
- Presence of addiction in one or both parents.
- Adverse childhood experiences.
- Poor parental or guardian relationships during childhood.

Recent years have seen an increase in the occurrence of new behavioural addictions, which are no longer associated with the use of

Sex addiction spectrum, risk factors and presenting signs

psychoactive substances but instead with the repetition of compulsive behaviours that cause emotional distress and suffering in the addict as well as in their family. In my practise, I've noticed a rise in patients who come to therapy for problems like a lack of intimacy, relationship conflict, poor parenting, job dissatisfaction, depression, anger issues and so on, only to find out after further investigation that the real problem is one partner's secretive compulsive sexual behaviour, which has affected every other aspect of their family system. This is not to imply that sex addiction is a brand-new form of brain disease or addiction, just that we are better able to identify and assess it now.

Sex addiction is the beast of all addictions and a well-kept secret. People can hide their behaviour for years without anybody detecting it while they keep ramping up their addiction, just like a heroin or ice junkie who needs more and more to reach arousal.

Unlike alcohol and substance addiction - which can be clearly detected from observing certain behaviours; gambling - which can be detected from missing money; eating disorders- which can be detected from weight fluctuation, sex addiction does not have any obvious signs unless someone has experienced them before or is trained to recognise them.

It can persist for a long time without being noticed. I frequently see betrayed partners who have been traumatised by the experience and who find it difficult to believe that their partners have been engaging in these illicit behaviours for such long periods.

They frequently say things like:

- I feel like a fool.
- I'm an intelligent person, so what does it say about me that he's been doing this for so long without my knowledge?

- He's not that kind of person, and he's usually around, so when did he have time?
- But he is so shy and never even flirts.
- He is not even tech savvy.
- Although he wasn't always fully present or a good listener or intimate, I thought he was my best friend.
- He is such a fantastic father.

I always respond that sex addiction is about maintaining a false persona, deception, and a double life in order to feed their addiction, just like other addictions. The other hidden personality surfaces and takes charge when the person needs their fix. Once the brain has produced the required amount of dopamine and they have eventually engaged in sexual behaviour, they can swiftly revert to their former roles as a loving parent, dependable professional and loyal partner..

According to the results of the research I conducted in 2021, every single sex addict man was actively engaging in their addiction years before entering their primary romantic relationships. Sex addiction always exists before and predates an intimate relationship, so the partners cannot be held responsible for causing it. NEVER. They get into a relationship with someone who brings in a wicked and invisible mistress. Since compulsive sexual behaviours begin when the brain is underdeveloped in early life and quickly become conditioned and driven to sustain them in order to experience the addictive dopamine rushes, no one wakes up as an adult and becomes a sex addict.

It's vital to keep in mind that not everyone who drinks alcohol becomes an alcoholic, and not every young person who engages in sexual behaviour becomes a sex addict. However, sex addiction is one of the rapidly spreading and well-hidden pandemics with a tsunami of negative effects on individuals and their interpersonal relationships

Sex addiction spectrum, risk factors and presenting signs

as a result of the accessibility, affordability, normalisation and availability of porn and other sexually explicit material and activities.

The sex addicts are individuals susceptible to this condition and have undergone some hardships and traumatic early life incidents or have been exposed to some kind of sexual experience, including seeing sexual activities or sexual images.

Engaging in fantasies, viewing pornographic imagery, and masturbating begin very early in life as a self-soothing technique. Eventually, these maladaptive soothing tools turn into numbing agents and regular conducts that drives the sex addict to seek for ever more sexual release in order to function on a daily basis. Sex addiction is closely linked to self-loathing, perpetuating the challenges in both personal and interpersonal relationships.

The intimate partner needs to improve their knowledge and become skilled in order to recognise the warning signs, which may include:

- Lack of presence and self-awareness.
- Lack of intimacy or empathy.
- Inability to express or share feelings.
- Poor listening skills
- Lying, deception or twisting the truth.
- Blame shifting, gaslighting, and manipulative behaviours.
- Spending excessive time on their phone or social media.
- Taking their phone into the shower or toilet.
- Constantly changing the passwords on their digital devices.
- People-watching.
- Either too much hypersexuality with the partner or very infrequent sexual intimacy.
- Lack of concentration and focus at work or home.

- Going to bed later than the partner and staying up late.
- Sexualizing language.
- Flirting.
- Poor financial and money management skills.
- When confronted by the hurt partner about improper flirtation, language, or behaviour, they quickly flip the situation around and blame and berate the partner.
- Defensiveness, stone walling or an angry outburst if confronted.
- Lack of deep and meaningful friendships, especially with those of the same sex.
- People pleasers and approval seekers.

According to Pornhub, the leading free porn site in the world, the consumption of pornography and viewing sexually explicit content has surged globally since March 2020, during the shutdown period. For example, in Australia, there has been an increase in visits to such pornography sites with a booming sex industry in this region.

The phrase "new addictions" has recently come into usage to describe addictions that are behavioural as opposed to those brought on by the use of drugs and psychoactive substances. Compulsive sexual behaviours/sex addiction, pathological gambling, excessive shopping, internet addiction, and workaholism are some of the new addictions that are on the rise.

The condition known as sexual addiction is understood as an above-average sexual behaviour and defined by intrusive and compulsive sexual thoughts and fantasies that are linked to a loss of control over sexual activity that has detrimental effects on all aspects of life such as work, mood, and social interaction.

Sex addiction spectrum, risk factors and presenting signs

The cerebral reward system of the brain, which controls a person's patterns of cravings, pleasure and satisfaction, is altered because of this psycho-physio-pathological condition.

Sex addiction is defined as an intense and compulsive urge that changes the subject's state of consciousness to the point that they are unable to control their impulses.

Drug addicts experience tolerance, and an increased need of drugs, a phenomena, sex addicts also experience. As a result, they may feel the need to intensify or increase their sexual practise in order to sustain the desired effect. The result of which will be actual psychophysiological alterations, such as an increase in emotional discomfort and feeling anxious.

Masturbation and the consumption of pornographic material are not harmful habits as long as they don't interfere with a person's life, become compulsive, or take over their daily routine.

Sex addiction is characterised by a persistent and intense preoccupation with sexual fantasies, impulses, and behaviours that results in clinically significant distress or impairment in social, occupational, or other key areas. Sex addiction is also characterised by a recurrent inability to exert control over or cut down on the amount of time spent engaging in these behaviours in response to negative moods or stressful life events.

People that engage in problematic hypersexual conduct tend to be highly impulsive, cognitively inflexible, imprecise, emotionally uncontrollable, and overly concerned with sex.

Sex addicts actually have a tendency to be attracted to stimuli that are associated to addiction. Previous research on drug addictions suggests that an abnormal rise in motivation and attention to salient stimuli may transform addiction into a disinhibitory disorder and lead to a loss of control.

Sexual addiction is a problem that could get worse in today's culture. People are constantly exposed to sexual stimuli, making it quite simple to develop an addiction of this kind.

Websites containing explicit photos and videos, social media sites like Facebook, Instagram, and Snapchat, escort sites, games, and messaging applications are just a few of the things the internet has to offer.

Digital technologies have invaded all spheres of social, political, economic, and cultural life, changing interpersonal relationships, individual identities, and patterns of demand and supply.

Sexual practises have also undergone major alteration as a result of these shifts. People who, most likely, in the absence of hyper-stimulation would not have become addicted find that new forms of twisted fantasies and sexual imagination have infiltrated their minds and are endangering their real-world relationships. This is brought on by advancements in technology, the normalisation of sexual behaviour, and a lack of valuable information.

Impulsive motivations that aim to fill emptiness and boredom drive sex addiction. But after the sexual act is over, the related reward circuit ends, and the same negative emotions like anxiety and depression return and are made worse by a strong sense of guilt.

Sex addiction is a disorder of the brain that affects not only the individual but also our society. Sex addiction is becoming more prevalent as a result of the normalisation of sexual behaviour and the ease with which it may be concealed. Nearly everyone has some connection to or knowledge of a sex addict. I frequently hear the same thing from betrayed partners:

'Why do the revelations about my partner make me feel so devastated? Until it happened to me I assumed that everyone was masturbating and watching porn. That appeared normal to me.'

I tell them that normal doesn't make it optimal. The majority of betrayed partners I meet are completely unaware of what is happening in the massage parlours that are springing up everywhere or at strip clubs. One woman admitted that she felt foolish for even considering taking her spouse to a strip club for entertainment. She had no idea that he had visited frequently and had even paid to have sex with a few of the strippers without her knowledge. In addition, her husband claimed that his weak back was to blame after she discovered some receipts from a massage parlour. He acknowledged during the polygraph test that, in order to alleviate her suspicions, he would always make cash payments whenever he visited such locations following that exposure. A few years prior, when they sought marital counselling, their therapist had advised her to be more daring in the bedroom but failed to assess further for potential sex addiction. Because of this, the unwary partner believed that inviting him to a strip club or watching porn together would be just what they needed to rekindle their romance. This narrative serves as an example of how manipulative and deceitful sex addicts can be in order to keep fuelling their addiction.

If you are the partner of a sex addict, please keep in mind that there is nothing you can do to fulfil his compulsive sexual behaviour. His insatiable needs cannot be satiated by any amount of sex. His primary issue isn't a lack of sex, a lack of the kind of sex he desires (some sex addicts can pressure their partners into anal sex or other sexual practises that the partner doesn't feel comfortable with), or anything else you might do to cure him. You cannot cure his condition because you did not cause it. His addiction originates in his brain rather than his genitalia. Instead of more particular types of sex, he needs detoxification and recovery from his addiction.

Porn and its link to SA

A type of sexual addiction known as porn addiction is characterised by uncontrollable levels of preoccupation and compulsivity. According to research, the majority of people who self-identify as having an addiction to or a compulsive interest in pornography today spend at least 11 or 12 hours per week watching (and typically masturbating to) porn that they access via their computer, laptop, tablet, smartphone, or other devices. It is important to note that the availability of pornography and other sexually explicit content around-the-clock thanks to technology has led to some users engaging in their sexual compulsive behaviours for far longer periods of time than the stated 11–12 hours per week.

People who are compulsively or addictively interested in pornography feel compelled to view porn. Over time, they begin to plan their life around porn. Important relationships, pursuits, and obligations can all be partially or entirely neglected as a result of a compulsive porn use. Porn addicts spend excessive amounts of time finding porn, watching porn, and compiling their collection. Frequently, when feeling guilty or repentant, they would promise themselves, *this is the last time I'm using pornography,* but are soon back to repeating the behaviour.

They occasionally feel good about purging their entire collection of porn. But when their pink cloud ultimately goes away, they regret

Sex addiction spectrum, risk factors and presenting signs

the deletion and hastily reassemble their collection. Many people often go through the delete-reassemble cycle repeatedly.

The following are typical indications that a user's casual porn consumption has become troublesome for them:

- Usage of pornography that has not stopped despite consequences or commitments to oneself or others to do so.
- Increasing amounts of time spent watching porn and difficulties limiting that.
- Time wasted searching for, organising, and watching porn.
- Excessive masturbation that causes cuts or injuries.
- Watching increasing numbers of outrageous pornographic material.
- Lying, hiding information, and minimising the type and volume of pornographic use.
- Irritation or anger when urged to quit watching porn.
- Diminished or absent interest in sex and intimacy in real life.
- Difficulty to reach orgasm, delayed ejaculation, and erectile dysfunction.
- Turning to porn to deal with uncomfortable feelings.
- Relationship difficulties.
- Increasing the intensity of or the violence in the pornographic content

Sadly, those who battle with pornography are frequently hesitant to ask for treatment because they do not perceive their solo sexual practises as the primary reason of their dissatisfaction. And when they do, they don't actually seek help for the porn problem but rather for symptoms associated to it including anxiety, loneliness, and relationship issues.

Porn addiction can disrupt relationships and generate conflict because excessive pornography viewing can make a person prefer porn and screen intimacy to true intimate connections. Watching porn helps people forget about their relationship problems, creating a loop that could be destructive.

For example, in the US and Australia, most men (64–70%) consume pornography on a regular basis. This has significantly affected intimate partners' overall wellness and relationship satisfaction.

Many people receive therapy for lengthy periods of time without ever mentioning or even being questioned about masturbation or pornography. Either the patient is too ashamed to discuss their porn use, they fail to perceive the connection between their addiction and their difficulties, or the therapist lacks the expertise to make the appropriate assessment. Because of this, their primary issue remains unresolved and hidden.

The use of pornography within a relationship is frequently justified as being helpful in enhancing sexual arousal or increasing sexual satisfaction for both partners. However, based on evidence only less than 10% use pornography within a romantic relationship and 90% use it alone and in secret. In turn, pornography consumption has been found to reduce the levels of commitment in a relationship for both men and women.

Some people believe the impacts on intimate relationships would be less severe if compulsive sexual behaviours are restricted to porn and masturbation without indulging in any physical infidelities. This presumption has quickly been challenged by research showing that, despite the absence of any physical infidelity, all intimate partners of such individuals had similar betrayal trauma, severe emotional reactions and relational trust and satisfaction are substantially

Sex addiction spectrum, risk factors and presenting signs

harmed. In addition, research on porn addiction has found that it can lead to feelings of doubt about the relationship as well as anxiety, resentment, trauma, rejection, isolation, shame, and a sense of abandonment and betrayal in intimate partners (See figure 1). Compulsive consumption of pornography can contribute to a careless attitude towards sexual behaviours and has been linked to a high rate of infidelity in relationships.

Figure 1 illustrates the multifaceted negative impacts that compulsive pornography use can have on intimate partner wellbeing.

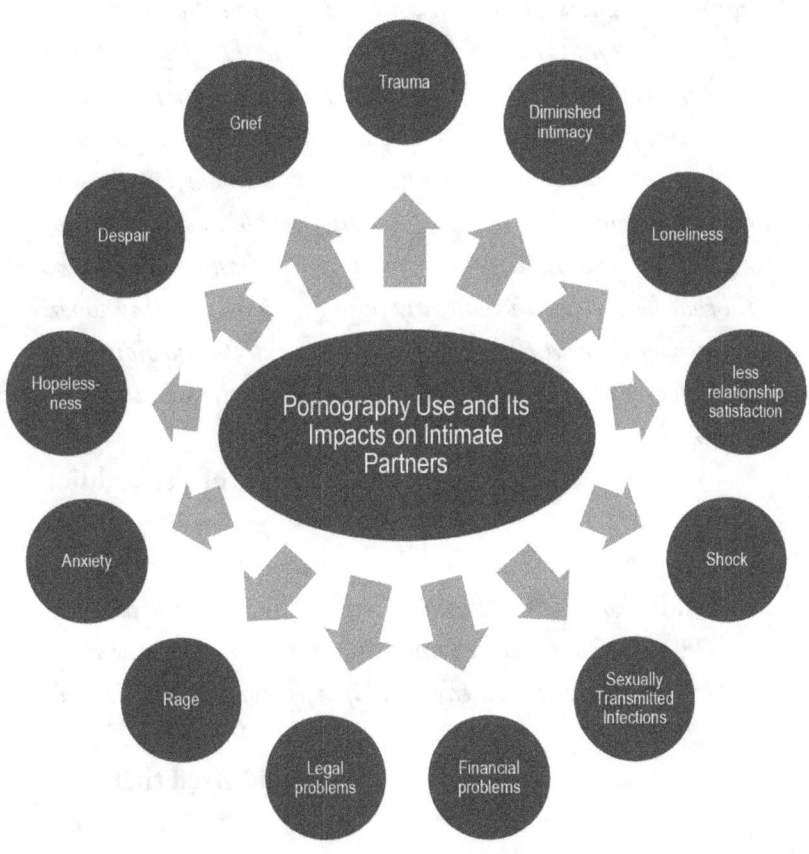

I had been married to my husband for ten years, with a young child together. At the beginning of our relationship, I suspected his pornography consumption. However, much later I found out about his secretive masturbation, excessive preoccupation with sex, and fantasies. Pre discovery he frequently would accuse me of depriving him of the amount or type of sex he desired. He also told me that he watched porn to spice up our sex life. Although deep down I didn't like it I didn't have a clue how much he was watching it. To be honest, I did not understand the full extent or seriousness of his sex addiction until recently. I acknowledge that I was unaware of SA before making my initial discovery. I found a hidden SIM card and various email addresses he had used to communicate with other people. He confessed that in order to support his habits, money had been routinely taken out of our bank accounts. I later learned that he had engaged in a variety of risky sexual behaviours, including paying for sex, having impromptu hook-ups, following people on social media, and having unprotected sex with complete strangers. Later, he said that he had begun watching porn and masturbating when he was young, and that his compulsive sexual behaviour had gotten worse over time and throughout the entire length of our relationship.

Karen, wife of a sex addict

I wish society as a whole was more conscious of the harm caused by porn. In movies and television shows, it is portrayed as being perfectly acceptable, normal and something that everyone does. People joke about it and say it as if it is normal, but it isn't because it is harmful.

Peter, licensed therapist

Sex addiction spectrum, risk factors and presenting signs

Please be aware, as a betrayed partner, that your sex addict mate may not even be engaging in much sex but that their sexual preoccupation and the chatter in their head may rule their interactions, their thoughts, and their lives. They may use these behaviours and preoccupations to numb and escape instead of deepening and appreciating them.

CHAPTER 2

Living with a sex addict

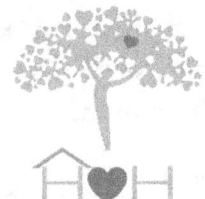

Sex addiction is a major problem that frequently starts before your romantic relationship does. Although the causes of someone being addicted can be complex, the effects are startlingly straightforward: this addiction hurts all parties involved.

Along with the complicated problems that contribute to compulsive behaviour, a spouse faces particular difficulties when sexual addiction is suspected or confirmed. As a betrayed partner when exposed to your spouse's addiction you could find yourself wondering, *How did I not see this coming?* or *How can I live with an addict?*

The majority of addictions are destructive to relationships because the partner who is pursuing the addiction typically makes the other partner feel abandoned or abused. Most partners find it particularly difficult to live with a sex addict because the condition directly affects a number of powerful emotions, including jealousy and the exclusivity and sacredness of intimacy.

Sex addicts find it difficult or impossible to stay faithful or honest to their partners, even when they are aware that their pursuit of sex would likely involve neglect, lying, spending money carelessly, and a high risk of getting sexually transmitted disorders or causing unplanned pregnancies.

Any of the aforementioned factors, such as feelings of loneliness, depression, betrayal, shame, and resentment, could cause your sex addict partner a great deal of suffering. As a result, the relationship could then further deteriorate, long before the partner of a sex addict is aware of what is happening in the secretive world of the addict.

Even the best intentions and sympathy can be tested to the breaking point in relationships with sex addicts, which typically result in pain and regret on both sides.

You may have gone through both or just one of the following with your sex addict partner. Which of the following is relevant to your relationship?

In the early stages of a relationship, partners of sex addicts frequently spend a lot of time believing that something is wrong with them if they are unable to meet their partner's demands in this area. The regularity with which sex is demanded and the potential lack of intimacy in the sexual experience can overwhelm someone who is dating or married to a sex addict. Most partners of sex addicts will admit that even if they enjoyed having sex with them, they rarely felt connected while doing so:

- *I felt something wasn't right but couldn't put my finger on it.*
- *I blamed myself for my busy schedule with my children, my weight gain.*

On the other hand, the sex addict may express little to no desire in having sex with their real partner and may excuse this behaviour by blaming their busy schedules, demanding jobs, or exhaustion. In actuality, compulsive sexual behaviours smother the pleasure, desire, and delight of engaging in sex with a real partner.

> *We had just been married a few years when I believed we needed to rekindle our sex because he didn't seem content or close to me. To improve myself, I started reading books and seeking counselling. I believed I was entirely to blame, yet it never worked... To satisfy his expectations, there was a time when I somewhat increased my hypersexuality, and that is when I began to feel like a pincushion. Looking back, I can say that time traumatised me even more and made me feel very ashamed and unworthy. Although it didn't strengthen our bond, it did make me feel awful about my marriage and myself.*
> **Anne, betrayed partner**

Anxiety, low self-esteem, guilt, embarrassment, and many other emotions might result from believing that you can't sexually please your partner. Additionally, you could worry about your partner's loyalty or potential STD exposure.

A person with a sex addiction experiences the same level of urgency to use their drug of choice (sexual release) as a person with a heroin addiction. The urges are powerful and challenging to resist.

I finally agreed to a threesome because of his persuasiveness and cunning. He destroyed my integrity and morals, and to be very honest, I don't know how I allowed myself to get to that point. I was in a bad place and wanted for us to be a family after giving birth to my second daughter. Even worse, he convinced me that it was all about him being more willing to have sex with me, giving me the pleasure I deserved and not about him. He led me to feel that I had the power to decide who to invite in. To say that I experienced multiple panic attacks while experiencing that awful threesome act would be an understatement. I started crying and then locked myself in the bathroom. After learning about his severe sex addiction, I came to understand that, after our threesome failed, he had other secret encounters with that woman. I find it shocking that he frequently accused me of being boring sexually. He made me feel flawed and unattractive. I'm upset with myself for being so foolish as to let him treat me that way. I had no idea what sex addiction even was. Now that I know the actual extent of his disease, I am receiving extensive counselling, taking anti-anxiety medicine, sleeping pills, and alcohol to numb the agonising sting of betrayal. I'm a mess.

Patricia, partner of a sex addict

Most sex addicts actually need and want intensely intimate relationships with their partners, but they are also afraid and unable of giving or receiving it. They often become romantically distant from their relationships as a result of this. Instead, these individuals frequently struggle with intimacy because they get a false sense of safe intimacy from pornography, masturbation, or other compulsive sexual activities. This false sense of safety is perceived because there is frequently no need for attachment or requirements to be emotionally invested. It becomes safer for them to act out with sex workers or pornographic material rather than having to be intimate and honest with their partners.

As a partner of a sex addict, keep in mind that sex addiction has nothing to do with you or your sexual conduct and everything to do with his brain chemical dependency. They would have done exactly what they have done regardless of who you were. A growing number of famous couples are coming forward to acknowledge that their partners are sex addicts. These are frequently gorgeous individuals who are in excellent shape and who have achieved great success, but their sex addict partners have betrayed them in a manner not unlike your partner has. Your ability to satisfy your partner's sexual desires has absolutely no bearing on a person's ability to develop a sex addiction. The problem with sex addiction is the way it's used to escape loneliness, emotional pain, unworthiness, shame, and issues with attachment and intimacy dysfunction. The majority of betrayed partners encounter their sex addict partner's anger, depression, lack of empathy, avoidance of uncomfortable emotions, and defensive attitudes before discovery or disclosure but are unaware of the causes of such behaviours. Research has also demonstrated a link between depression, aggression, and rage and a higher risk of addiction, including sex addiction.

If you have been in a relationship with a sex addict, you have undoubtedly witnessed their **passive aggression.** Passive aggression is when someone feels furious but avoids confrontation by acting out in passive ways, such as giving others the quiet treatment or pretending everything is fine when it isn't.

Alternatively, you may have experienced their **open aggression.** Open aggression which is overt hostility results from a desire to be in control. In this type of anger, the sex addict may lose control and become physically or verbally violent and aggressive out of feelings of rage or shame. As a means of taking control, they may bully, shout, threaten with blackmail, or criticise others.

Their **lack or complete absence of empathy** is another noted characteristic shortcoming of most sex addicts. Empathy, or the capacity to recognise, comprehend, and analyse another person's feelings, is such an important ability. Without empathy, a sex addict lacks the ability to put oneself in another person's shoes and cares nothing about how their actions can hurt someone else. Empathy is a learned skill and can be cultivated during sex addiction recovery. Many sex addicts lack this ability inherently, but it can be developed and learned intentionally over time. Though it can be a sign of borderline personality disorder and narcissistic tendencies, which are present in certain sex addicts, if a person never acquires the skill of empathy.

Other behavioural dysfunctions frequently observed in sex addicts include **avoidance** and **repression**. Avoidance is the act of avoiding specific situations, people, objects, places, and in the context of sex addiction, unpleasant emotions and conflicts. This avoidance may be driven by fear of the undesirable results or by unpleasant and anxious feelings associated with them. It is a dysfunctional coping strategy for managing anxiety or a response to fear or shame. For instance, a sex addict typically participates in avoidance behaviours to avoid conflicts with a partner who challenges some of their choices or behaviours. These can involve leaving the house, giving silent treatment or simply walking away. They can continue their risky behaviour by avoiding these situations without having to deal with anxiety or the shame of doing so in front of their partners. Sex addicts are adept in repression of unpleasant feelings and actions, particularly those connected to their sexually acting out behaviours.

Repression is the unintended masking of painful memories, undesirable thoughts, or false beliefs. Repressing is meant to make these unpleasant experiences fully disappear. However, the memories, ideas, or convictions persist and suppression becomes depression. Additionally, suppression inadvertently impacts on how the sex addict acts around others, sparking anger or frustration and destroying relationships.

Another common trait seen in sex addicts is **defensiveness**. Defensiveness frequently stems from an effort to defend oneself against perceived threats. Many times, sex addicts (before recovery) use these psychological reactions unintentionally and do not deliberately choose to do so. Defensiveness provides the individuals with drug, alcohol or sex addiction with a means of avoiding problems, resisting change, and rationalising unreasonable behaviour. When this occurs, sex addicts often become argumentative in their views and attitudes and refuse to consider the viewpoint of another person. They frequently reverse the situation and accuse the other party of making them feel that way. A sex addict may become defensive when confronted about questionable behaviours because they fear being rejected, feel like failures, abandoned, losing control or shamed. The goal of defensive responses is to divert the sex addict's attention away from their painful emotions and shame. Whether they realise it or not, the aim is to attract attention to the partner's flaws so that they feel better about themselves at the time.

Knowing how your partner might engage in defensiveness is important if you are a partner of a sex addict.

- They stop paying attention or listening to the partner.
- Giving the partner the silent treatment or stone walling them which means being silent in response to their criticism.
- Provide justifications for whatever is being criticised.
- Place the blame on the partner.
- Make false accusations or lie.
- Attempt to minimise or rationalise their behaviour.
- Using deflection to void addressing the current issue by talking about the other person's past mistakes.
- Displaying righteous anger and acting as if the sex addict shouldn't be questioned about this for some reason.
- Try to convince the partner that their feelings are inappropriate.
- Using gaslighting as a way of denial or trickery to cast doubt on partner's sanity or memory. In order to accomplish this, the sex addict indicates that the partner is acting irrationally, crazy or not thinking straight.
- Agreeing with the criticism while simultaneously blaming the partner or crying in order to make the other person feel guilty and gain compassion. This is a deceptive manoeuvre used to stop further criticism.

Reasons for defensiveness in a sex addict partner:

- Creating the appearance of security as a response to feelings of insecurity or anxiety in order to feel more powerful and in control at the time.
- Fabricating a false sense of safety and security.
- An emotional reaction to childhood maltreatment or other traumatic events.
- Response to anxiety, unworthiness or an inability to speak up for oneself.
- A reaction to guilt or shame.
- Diverting attention from a deception.
- Retaliation for what is believed to be a character or behaviour attack.
- Avoiding disagreement or conflict.
- Refusal to acknowledge mistakes or shortcomings.
- Inability to constructively respond to criticism.
- A manifestation of a mental health disorder or addiction.
- A learned behaviour.

Sex addicts have a tendency to **gaslight** others. Gaslighting is a form of psychological abuse where a sex addict manipulates their partner into questioning their own judgement or even their sanity. It is not only sociopaths and psychopaths that are capable of this disturbing method of manipulation. In relationships where addiction is prevalent, gaslighting is a common occurrence. Gaslighting is therefore a phenomenon that sex addicts' partners experience rather regularly. This kind of infidelity-related sex addiction behaviour is something I commonly see in my clinical work. A sex addict will try to trick their partner into believing that they are the problem, that they are suspicious, and that they are looking for something that isn't there. In these situations, the unfaithful partner generally rejects the betrayed partner's intuition and reality for years while steadfastly insisting that they haven't had sex with anyone else and that the worried partner is just being unduly watchful, distrusting, and unfair. Over time, the betrayed partners start to distrust their ability to perceive reality, and they start to self-gaslight by feeling guilty and unjustified for their suspicions and instead believe the lies that the sex addict partner tells them.

Gaslighting occurs repeatedly over an extended period of time. It perpetuates betrayal trauma and results in chronic trauma. As a result, individuals who have been gaslighted frequently exhibit rage, emotional instability and fear.

In most cases, the challenge for the victim (betrayed partner) is that abuse takes place in a relationship that also has other, more positive aspects that might mask or overpower the abuse's true significance and impact. PTSD, anxiety disorders, depression, and other conditions have all been linked to chronic betrayal trauma behaviours such as gaslighting. The most intense agony a betrayed partner experiences is not from a specific sexual act that the sex addict has engaged in, but rather from the ongoing lies, denial of partner's reality, and gaslighting.

A complicated, multifaceted emotion that has been described as a combination of rage, fear, disgust, and disappointment is **resentment.** Several psychologists classify it as a mood or a secondary emotion with cognitive components. Resentment has the potential to be one of the strongest unpleasant feelings seen in the majority of sex addicts. Resentment naturally carries a sense of unfairness (from slight to extreme) as well as a strong defence against unfair people, organizations, or circumstances.

The emotion of resentment can be described as a silent angry voice because the person is made to accept something they do not like. For a number of reasons, many if not all addicts experience resentment. Perhaps they are frustrated with their current living condition, the mistakes they made, or the addiction itself. Resentment never appears on its own; it is always accompanied by its ugly sibling, entitlement. Together, they benefit the sex addict because when they show up, the addict frequently ends up receiving their fix through acting out.

This negative emotion leads to a secondary benefit for the addict; as a result, it is entwined with the current addiction cycle and keeps the addict in their active addiction pattern. Let me explain. Resentments are hazardous because they feed the entitlement of sex addicts, enabling them to continue their addictive behaviours while justifying their actions. In other words, individuals can feed the entitled mindset and continue to act out as long as they can persuade themselves to hold on to resentment. Because they lack emotional intelligence and empathy before getting sober, sex addicts see themselves as victims and blame their partners for their own compulsive behaviours.

They frequently believe or make up stories such…

- If she didn't nag so much
- If she gave me enough sex, or the kind of sex I deserve
- If she lost weight, etc.

…I wouldn't need to turn elsewhere to satiate my own sexual demands.

These misguided beliefs breed resentment, which makes it easier for individuals to distance themselves from their partners and feel entitled to engage in compulsive sexual behaviours while disregarding the repercussions.

If resentment is not regularly addressed throughout the recovery process, it will impede, and harm the healing process, and prevent the restoration of relationships.

Signs of Resentment in your sex addict partner:

The inability to let go or forgive.

Unprocessed negative emotions that recur, including annoyance, animosity, anger, bitterness, and unease.

Failure to stop thinking about an unfortunate **event.**

Remorse or feelings of shame and regret (self-resentment).

Avoidance based on fear. When a sex addict is resentful, certain persons or situations may trigger unwanted memories of past offenses. As a result, they can opt to avoid situations or individuals that give them this feeling. Addicts routinely take such actions to protect their own safety and concerns.

Dysfunctional relationship skills. Changes in the relationship may result from resentment. Holding grudges and engaging in passive-aggressive behaviour are two ways some people cope with resentment.

Feeling inadequate or insignificant. **Expecting** recognition for something while not getting it. Alternatively, interacting with people or situations that bring up unpleasant emotions from the past can make the addict feel unimportant or invisible. When this happens, buried feelings of bitterness and resentment may reawaken and grow.

Having trouble letting go. In other cases, the addict may find it difficult to let go of their rage due to resentment. Such people could even have a strong desire for vengeance. Their mental health suffers as a result of holding onto such an extreme amount of negativity.

A neglected aspect of a recovering addict's life is **entitlement**. It is evidently a significant factor in the breakdown and derailment of many addicts who are controlled by their narcissistic wound. It could be obvious, like a bulging black eye, or commonly subtle and undetectable, like a blind spot. I've seen it in all sex addicts I have treated and I have come to believe that sex addiction is an addiction to feeling entitled, an addiction to expecting something for nothing. This maladaptive behaviour is another survival mechanism and has been identified throughout the period of sex addiction.

First, due to the high expectations of their partner and lack of reciprocation, addicts who are still in the active addiction phase typically act in this manner. They feel justifiable in brazenly betraying their partners through evasive compulsive behaviours while holding them responsible for a majority of relational dysfunctions. Second, many recovering sex addicts still have delusions and demand quick healing and forgiveness from their partners while making very little progress in their actual recovery. These people frequently act like victims and whine when things aren't going their way.

The easiest place for addicts to revert to is victim state. This has been their default stance throughout their lives to soothe their guilt and shame and hold others responsible for their own failings. It is fuelled by deprivation, which is often a lack caused on by unfulfilled emotional needs. Most addicts were never taught how to handle their emotional needs in a healthy way. They frequently exhibit an emotional child mind attitude. Children always feel like victims and demand that adults make them feel better and take responsibility for their well-being. They present themselves as victims and attribute their problems to other people or outside forces. A sense of entitlement is prone to emerge in someone who frequently feels as though terrible things are happening to them. They believe they are entitled to everything and that it is the obligation of other people to make their lives better. In my practise, I frequently encounter recovering sex addicts who put very little effort into their sobriety and recovery and invariably attribute their own inadequacies to a lack of time, children, an uncooperative partner, or ineffective therapy.

People who feel entitled frequently have a self-centred attitude on life and show little consideration for how their actions affect other people—they lack empathy. An excessive case of entitlement could be a sign of a personality disorder such as narcissistic personality disorder or antisocial personality disorder. The opposite of gratitude is a sense of entitlement, which leads sex addicts to constantly dwell on their misfortunes rather than their blessings. They do not express gratitude for their privileges. A person who feels entitled cannot express thanks or other forms of appreciation for what they have. They don't value anything because they believe they should have everything, which causes them to value nothing.

When having a sense of entitlement, anything that challenges someone's sense of superiority over others is received with fury and defensiveness. A vicious loop results in the more they are hampered by others and society norms, the more resentful they become about these perceived injustices. Studies have shown that resentment and entitlement can be damaging. People who are resentful and entitled are more prone to experience ongoing disappointment, unmet expectations, and addictive behaviour patterns that put them and those around them in harm.

This is how a sex addict's brain justifies acting out sexually:

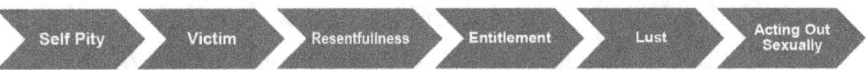

Another flaw in sex addicts is their need for **external approval,** which drives them to great lengths to appease others in order to receive it. They are always looking to others for admiration and praise. An attitude of entitlement commonly coexists with narcissistic tendencies. Sex addicts who are only concerned with what makes them feel good about themselves are often highly reliant on the attention and affirmation of others. This is yet another maladaptive survival mechanism. On the one hand, this results from a safety seeking desire and from the desire to perceive the environment and the people in it as safe. On the other side, they are attempting to satisfy their own emotional demands and requirements for external approval. To put it another way, this is an egocentric characteristic that makes it all about oneself. Lack of self-worth is the root cause of approval seeking tendencies, which can be exacerbated by a number of factors, including an addict's natural personality as well as external influences like childhood, the family structure, culture, education, and past life experiences. People who engage in approval-seeking behaviours usually suffer from low self-confidence and self-esteem.

For some people, this way of thinking might appear so natural that it becomes their default way of thinking.

You might have noticed the following approval seeking behaviours in your sex addict partner:

- Having trouble accepting Difference. Are they overly sensitive to dispute or do they take it personally when someone disagrees with them?
- In response to criticism, they may change their opinions. How do they react when someone disagrees with them after they express their viewpoint on a subject (whether serious or not)? Do they stand by their position or do they start to compromise on their principles and shape their thoughts to more closely resemble the other person's?
- Because they lack self-confidence, addicts who engage in approval-seeking behaviour frequently modify their thoughts depending on who they are speaking to. They worry that their opinions are incorrect and don't want to alienate people by holding a different opinion.
- This does not apply to intimate partners. They rarely conform to their opinions because of the fabricated resentment they harbour for their intimate partners (more of this later).
- They say yes when they mean no? When asked to do something, do they say yes even though they would prefer to say no out of fear of being rejected? As a result, they may feel exhausted, apprehensive, or even unhappy. They might also harbour grudges against the people and events surrounding that involvement.

- When they don't want to, they still appease people.
- Do they occasionally give the impression that they agree with someone verbally or nonverbally even though they don't? This is typically an automatic reaction that results from low self-esteem, and fear of conflict and rejection.
- Claiming to understand or be knowledgeable about something when they are merely pretending to do so. There are times when sex addicts may feel as though they are the only one who doesn't understand a notion or idea. They can begin to question their understanding of the topic or worry that they lack a particular talent as a result. In that instance, the sex addict will lie instead of seeking an explanation.

Another serious issue with sex addicts is their **lack of self-awareness.**

The capacity to observe oneself clearly and objectively through reflection and observation is known as self-awareness. Before beginning an effective recovery process, sex addicts lack emotional intelligence, which has a direct relationship to self-awareness.

The capacity to appropriately regulate and understand one's own feelings and those of others (empathy) is known as emotional intelligence. It's a necessary social talent for effective performance, healthy conflict resolution, expressing feelings and needs, meaningful interactions with others, better mental health and effective communication. The good news is that emotional intelligence can be improved and grown over time. However, it necessitates self-improvement that is constant and intentional. Self-awareness and emotional intelligence are interrelated and developing either will enhance the other. The ability to evaluate oneself or be self-aware, which is the capacity to pay attention to one's inner self, is made possible for sex addicts by developing emotional intelligence. For a recovering sex addict to practise self-control, self-awareness is a critical ability since it enables them to evaluate their choices and choose whether they are the best ones to help them achieve their goals.

> **You may notice your partner's increased self-awareness during recovery when:**
>
> - They may become more assertive, more accepting, and more motivated to pursue transformative change and positive self-development.
> - They are able to exercise self-control, think critically, work creatively and productively, feel grateful for their recovery work, and have a healthy sense of self-worth.
> - They make better decisions.
> - Self-awareness can improve a person's performance at work, communication skills, and interpersonal relationships.
> - Your partner is engaging in recovery because they want to, not because they feel they have to because they are now fully aware of the wide-ranging implications.
> - Your partner is aware of their own triggers and manages them to avoid placing themselves in circumstances where they might succumb to temptation.
> - Your partner is empathetic towards you and your feelings, and rather than disregarding them, they strive to comfort and support you. Due to their self-awareness, they choose to sit in your emotions rather

- than turning it into a personal attack and making it about themselves.
- Your partner is attuned with their own uncomfortable emotions and is addressing them in a wholesome manner.
- Before speaking or acting compulsively, your partner is more likely to press their inner pause button.

The facts about your life with a sex addict partner:

Your suspicions were always justified and true
If you have had past unresolved conflicts with your partner, it's normal to downplay or minimise your relationship's sense of distance. Certain interpersonal attachment patterns clearly increase unreasonable and unrealistic jealousy behaviours. You can relax knowing that you were not crazy or unreasonable for feeling the way you did now that you are aware of the truth regarding his double life. Because, when there are overt signals of inappropriate sexual behaviour or language, it usually signifies there is a deeper problem.

Unfortunately, when presented with circumstantial proof, few sex addicts acknowledge to having a problem. An addict typically needs to be caught before they admit they have a problem and agree to get therapy.

You are not to blame for his sex addiction
It's not your fault that your partner has a sex addiction. Don't let individuals who lack education or knowledge try to convince you otherwise. The decision to engage in sexual behaviour is one that is entirely up to the individual. Deviant sexual behaviour is almost always decided upon and started before you meet your partner.

This has nothing to do with your sexual performance, age, or body shape. This has to do with your partner's inability to foster intimacy and connection. Undoubtedly, there are relationship dysfunctions that need to be addressed because by choosing to pursue comfort, affection, and pleasure elsewhere, your partner has left little opportunity for relationship issues to improve and has instead made them worse. Remember that no partner can compete with or overcome another person's addiction unless the addicted individual agrees to remove the third wheel (addiction) from the relationship. Accepting responsibility for your partner's choices and addiction is the worst thing you can do. You are however, solely accountable for your own healing.

It is common for betrayal trauma responses to be devastating and for you to feel stuck
While it may seem unfair, the truth is that, even if it's not your fault, your partner's sexual decisions have a significant and direct impact on you. In my recent research on Australian intimate partners of sex addicts, I discovered that everyone experienced a variety of detrimental side effects as a result of betrayal trauma after learning that their partner had engaged in compulsive sexual behaviour. Loss of self-esteem, panic attacks, suicidal thoughts, self-harm, anxiety, depression, despair, an inability to trust, loss of sexual freedom and satisfaction, uncertainty, and fear of the future are just a few of the harmful consequences. In addition, I discovered that a betrayed partner can get trapped in an agonizing emotional pendulum that alternates between a desire for connection with the sex addict partner and a simultaneous dread of it. Relatedly, a severe violation of trust is the fundamental aspect of betrayal. If it simply extinguished the love, the betrayal's pain would be trivial. But it's never really that easy. The real hurt of betrayal comes from the fact that love and affection frequently remain long after the harm has been done. It is similar to being forced to endure the pain of an injury that is not healable or

carriable. Being betrayed by someone you trusted and loved causes you to feel torn between love (desire for connection) and destruction (dread of connection) and unsure of which direction to take.

Moreover, my research found that intimate relationships hold certain values that build trust and security for partners. Whether contractually agreed to or not, it is generally expected that commitment and fidelity are essential to the wellbeing of an intimate relationship. Seeking and forming attachments in intimate relationships is one of the important developmental tasks. This appears to be the desired and ideal life sequence for most people. However, when this order is broken, oftentimes through the deception of sex addiction, the betrayed partners suffer negative emotional, physical, sexual, relational, and spiritual impacts. For a committed primary partner, betrayal can be traumatising because it erodes trust. Every area of the partners' existence and lives will be affected by the traumatic betrayal experiences that were triggered. Unaware of the reasons and circumstances surrounding these events, it sends the betrayed partner on a rollercoaster of emotions. The betrayed partner is unable to leave the relationship since they require the sex addict for emotional attachment and emotional survival because they recall the good moments and positives about them. However, the impact of the betrayal is so great that ongoing reminders and triggers of the events prevent the betrayed partner from feeling satisfied to continue the relationship. Consequently, if you first feel trapped in the relationship and unable to leave or remain there without feeling considerable suffering or experiencing perplexity, please know that this is a frequent side effect of betrayal trauma and that it will get better.

You matter, and so do your choices and experiences
You may go through a range of reactions when you first discover the extent of your partner's sexual misconduct, and you may find yourself experiencing an emotional roller coaster.

Some betrayed partners may stay in their relationships because they value forgiveness or because they uphold the idea of a relational covenant and its objectives. Some people may not feel true contentment because they find it difficult to accept their relationship as it is and are compelled to let go of their preconceived assumptions about its sincerity in light of the truth they have discovered. The discovery and disclosure are constant reminders of a murky history. The option to stay in a relationship seems to include giving up pride, self-respect, and dignity while also living in constant worry that their partner may engage in the same compulsive behaviours. However, while you are experiencing acute trauma, and trying to make sense of your experiences give yourself permission to not make a definite decision. It is not a good idea to base important decisions in life on the intense emotions you may be going through following discovery or disclosure.

To go past the grief's shock stage, give healing and time a chance to occur. It is essential to seek treatment from a betrayal trauma with a sex addiction specialist to successfully navigate through the complex grieving process. Always keep in mind that you can only heal what you let yourself feel.

Social isolation and false shame aren't yours to carry
Shame wants to make you feel inadequate and responsible for your partner's sexual dysfunction. Shame always seeks isolation and never facilitates your healing, integration, or healthy connections. The betrayed partner may mistakenly believe that they are an extension of their sex addict partners and accomplices in their actions due to certain cultural stigma, which results in false guilt, self-imposed isolation and shame. They frequently struggle to distinguish between the real and unreal parts of their lives and relationships with their partners. As a result, there is a lack of trust in both themselves and others, self-judgment for not seeing the behaviours sooner, which

makes them feel lonely and isolated and ashamed of themselves. Most of the impacted partners do not receive the proper support or aid, which adds to their suffering and bewilderment and makes them feel hopeless and as though society has failed and wronged them as well.

Once you realise that you are valuable and deserving of love and respect, you will be able to discern between your partner's conduct and how you feel about yourself. This will enable you to practise effective self-care, which will raise the possibility that many of your relationships can heal.

Gain control and reclaim your power

You have the power to decide whether to stay or leave the relationship, run or fight, establish boundaries, forgive, and find help for your healing process. Having choices will allow you to be more deliberate in your approach to life and social interactions. As unjust as it may seem, the truth is that your partner is a sex addict who committed all of the acts they did. It is what it is. If you try to invent an alternative reality or dispute what it is, you will only prolong your trauma. Some of your questions will never be resolved since there is no compelling answer that could alleviate the excruciating ache of betrayal without keeping you a helpless victim. You don't have to continue living like a victim while you're recovering, despite the fact that you were the victim of a betrayal of love and trust. You can develop the ability to control the choices you make in order to pursue health and quality of life. You will undoubtedly require a lot of support, resources, and motivation along the way, but as you make positive decisions to obtain the support you require for your healing, you'll discover the power you need for your family and for yourself. You may set boundaries, choose to forgive, and fight for restoration in healthy ways that promote healing, empowerment, and wholeness when you believe and feel that you are capable, valued, and powerful.

You are powerless over your partner's addiction
No matter how hard you try, you cannot change your partner. The only person you can change is yourself. Believing you can control your partner's behaviour by constant monitoring and threatening them will only increase your anxiety and harm your self-worth, boundaries, and health. Your boundaries, consequences and what you let your partner bring into the relationship are your only healthy defences.

There is nothing you can do but take care of yourself till the sex addict sincerely wants recovery for themselves. Despite the fact that you are helpless to address your partner's problem, your boundary should be that he must seek specialist counselling and recovery. Sending him to individual therapy will be a mistake if you plan to stay with him because joint counselling with a specialist is the only way for the two of you to heal, recover and possibly reconcile.

In my clinic, I frequently treat couples who have been receiving individual therapy for years with no progress. This is partially due to the fact that sex addicts are skilled at deceit and manipulation, and that when they seek therapy on their own, they lie, withhold information from the therapist, and maintain secrets. Another explanation is that since sex addiction is about dysfunctional intimacy, it is impossible for a sex addict to develop intimacy and empathy on their own or outside of a relationship restoration. According to research and my clinical experience, for the effective healing and recovery of both partners, individual therapy in combination with couple therapy in the same practise with the same therapist or therapists who collaborate with each other and are aligned is necessary.

Rebuilding a new relationship with the same partner after sex addiction is possible if the addict is committed to long-term behavioural change (solid sobriety) and maintaining their integrity while living authentically. If you decide to stay in your relationship with the addict, it will usually take some time before you are able to trust anything the addict says or does. The relational restoration is considerably more possible when you join them in their progress by also taking part in a process of recovery, healing, support, education, and self-examination.

Avoid rushing the forgiveness process
The partner's capacity for forgiveness is one of the biggest obstacles to mending a relationship that has been damaged by sexual addiction. Any prospect for reconciliation will be undermined by bitterness or retaliation. However, forgiveness is a process best served with lots of patience. Give yourself grace and time to walk the journey instead of rushing it or being rushed. This is especially true for people of faith who might feel pressured to forget and forgive quickly without giving themselves enough time to grieve and recover from their trauma. In my research on the intimate partners of sex addicts, I discovered that the majority of the betrayed partners lacked access to necessary information, validation, or a safe space within their religious communities. Instead, a demand for speedy forgiveness was felt by several.

It is crucial for healing and spiritual preservation to offer a safe community free from spiritual gaslighting and pressure to forgive quickly. Most affected partners still have a great deal of grieving to do, and forgiveness is not their first priority. On occasion, it might be difficult to refuse forgiveness when it is expected in specific social contexts. But do not submit to these religious or social norms as a betrayed partner. Don't anticipate that you will be able to forgive right away; you will know when you are ready. Some people may forgive quickly but you are unique, you may forgive your partner a little bit at the time and after your own trauma has stabilised. If so, that's fine. While forgiveness is not a refusal to accept the offence, one must first feel safe enough to assume a stance of peace towards the offender in order to truly forgive.

Not all boundary violations and unlimited chances to repent are grounds for forgiveness. It does not imply that the betrayal story should be forgotten.

CHAPTER 3

Your sex addict partner's intimacy dysfunction and anorexia makes you feel lonely

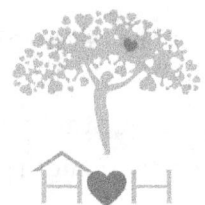

Dr. Doug Weiss, a pioneer in sex addiction therapy and partners' betrayal trauma recovery invented the phrase "intimacy anorexia" to describe how some sex addicts intentionally withhold emotionally, spiritually, and sexually from their partners. Problems surrounding emotional or physical intimacy can have a big impact on intimate relationships. And besides, to truly love someone is to desire to express your thoughts, feelings, and physical affection. Intimacy anorexia challenges frequently begin before discovery or disclosure and can be quite frustrating for an unsuspecting partner who constantly blames themselves for their partners' lack of connection. Intimacy anorexia frequently interferes with reconnection or full recovery during relationship restoration for many couples. The majority of sex addicts make slow progress in resolving their intimacy anorexia, which leaves their partners with more trauma and suffering. Dr Weiss found that the partner is severely harmed by this active withholding, which causes them emotional agony, grief, and anxiety. However, despite the pain they are causing, intimacy anorexics maintain their behaviour patterns. Ultimately, your relationship may start to feel hollow and unfulfilling when you love your anorexic partner but are unclear of whether they still feel the same way about you. You could worry that mutual intimacy will completely disappear as it begins to decline.

What are some ways your partner exhibits intimacy anorexia (Weiss, 2020)?

Staying busy – Intimacy anorexics are so busy and frequently find subtler ways to occupy themselves that they rarely have time for their partner. Being overly occupied at home could take the form of, playing with the kids alone or without the partner, doing chores, or working on solo tasks around the house. For many intimacy anorexics, technology is a dream come true since it gives them the impression that they are truly doing something or connecting with the visuals on a screen. Some people with intimacy anorexia purposefully avoid their partner by engaging in avoidant behaviours outside of the home. Anorexics who struggle with relationships can easily and convincingly defend their actions. Work is frequently cited by anorexic addicts as a good excuse for not spending time with their partners, giving them quality time, or even focusing on their own recovery.

Blaming you - The intimacy anorexic will hold their partner responsible for the relationship problems. Blame is nearly always a defining trait of intimacy anorexia. When a problem or issue arises in the relationship, the anorexic places the blame or responsibility for the problem on their partner rather than acknowledging their own involvement in the problem. You'll notice that intimacy anorexics constantly want to be right, which makes being flawed (careless, reckless, awful, etc.) unacceptable to discuss. Instead of examining their own behaviours, the sex addicts would blame their partner's actions for something they were not responsible for. Blame comprises misplaced resentment and a refusal to accept accountability for one's own actions.

Withholding Love - Intimacy anorexics actively withhold affection in the ways that their partners appreciate it. The anorexic frequently finds it challenging to understand the abstract nature of withholding love. Withholding love means not showing their spouse the affection they deserve or the way they desire. Despite the fact that we all desire love, we all have diverse experiences of it. Couples may desire lengthy walks, emotional conversations, or a meaningful note or present that expresses their feelings. Instead, anorexics will only give the kind of affection they are willing to give, regardless of what their partner wants.

Withholding Appreciation – Intimacy anorexics rarely compliment their partners in private. Refraining from giving praise is the same as keeping the partner in the dark about their excellent traits and how they have enhanced quality of life.

Withholding Sex - While some intimacy anorexics do engage in sex, the majority of them withhold that from their partners. Withholding sex is by far the most evident and, at the very least, the easiest to measure of all the behaviours that are signs of intimacy anorexia. Avoiding having sex, ruining sexual encounters, or failing to connect emotionally during sex are all examples of withholding sex. You may tell if you are the partner of an intimate anorexic by looking at when you last had sex.

Withholding Spiritually - Although intimacy addicts may be devout believers or even spiritual teachers, they rarely experience spiritual kinship at home. The partner is the only one to detect the spiritual withholding trait. Withholding spiritually means denying the partner a true sense of spiritual connection. This shows that there isn't any sincere spiritual behaviour between the couple and anyone else. Despite being a spiritual person, the anorexic lacks spiritual honesty with their partner. Instead, they act spiritually and religiously devoted to everyone else while denying the partner what they preach to others.

Inability to Share Feelings - The intimacy anorexic is unwilling or unable to express or disclose their emotions to their partner. The intimacy anorexic may find it frightening, challenging, or both to express their emotions in an authentic way. They might not be showing their partner the affection they know they prefer because they find it difficult or uncomfortable to communicate their feelings.

Criticism of the Partner - This criticism can be ongoing or unjustified.

This is another sign of intimacy anorexia with persistent or unjustified criticism that causes distance in the relationship. This can include using low-grade insults towards the partner, pointing out their mistakes, or simply routinely criticising their faulty views or choices. The unfounded criticism is largely unrelated to reality. If criticism is a deliberate tactic, intimacy anorexics will list their partner's flaws, weaknesses, and shortcomings far more quickly than they will list their partner's strengths.

Reacting with Silence, Anger, or Both- An intimacy anorexic may use silence, anger, or both to control their partner. The intimacy anorexia is not always characterised by silence or rage, but those who do so do so fiercely. Any use of rage or silence to distance oneself from, punish, or otherwise exert control over one's partner might be considered an intimacy anorexia trait. Some instances are extreme, such as when an intimacy anorexic refuses to communicate with their partner for days or weeks while they are still residing in the same home. The outburst of rage, which frequently stems from a minor offence, is a perfect method to alienate the partner and prevent them from opening up emotionally.

Money - The least frequent trait of intimacy anorexia is money, but when it does exist, it is extremely potent. Money will be used by the intimacy anorexic to control or shame the spouse. Those who use it do so with a strict hand. The majority of anorexics who use money to control or shame their partners do so by keeping them unaware of their finances, providing an allowance, forcing their spouse to ask for money, and preventing them from using a credit card online banking or chequebook. In this situation, the intimacy anorexic is fully permitted to spend money on whatever they want, but the partner is required to keep track of everything or is blamed for all expenditures, even reasonable ones.

Feeling like a Roommate - The partner of an intimacy anorexic feels more like a roommate than a partner. Intimacy anorexics typically display this because they avoid emotional connection. The feature that has been seen in the vast majority of intimacy anorexics who have been married or have had extended relationships can be summed up by the word 'roommate.'

Although the addict may seem self-centred and motivated by self-gratification, there are deeper core issues. Finding a way to have some satisfaction without having to undergo intense pain and anorexia are the main objectives for addicts and intimacy anorexics. Shame and sexual impulse control are always to blame. Additionally, it's the fear of being vulnerable or rejected. The same addicts will frequently feel incredibly needy and lonely while taking every precaution to avoid intimacy. Addicts occasionally recognise their want for connection; other times, they go their entire lives without experiencing close intimacy and are unsure of what they are missing. Then, isolation and loneliness may be used as a justification for engaging in sexual behaviours.

A sizable portion of sex addicts are unaware of their level of fear in intimate relationships. They most typically come from disconnected families where they had insufficient or inappropriate parental bonding. They unknowingly adopted a style of life that centres on avoiding intimacy and living in fear of connections. Many sex addicts use their compulsive acting out as a replacement for an intimate relationship. Their compulsive behaviours give off a false sense of intimacy. In fact, experiencing sexual fulfilment in what is thought to be a controlled situation reinforces it. Because the sex addict has complete control over the quantity of intimacy offered and received, it makes no emotional demands on the addict.

CHAPTER 4

Discovery & Disclosure

The addiction's discovery is typically a surprise. You may believe your life was going along fairly normally until you found out there is a huge amount of pornography on the computer or that the person you are with has had a completely hidden life you didn't know about.

Partners should take care of their own mental health because they can suffer greatly from having so many questions for which there aren't immediately apparent answers. When sexual addiction is first discovered, it can feel like an atomic explosion, bringing with it a unique set of problems and trauma to the relationship. To say that the shock of discovering in-person or online activities can be disastrous is an understatement.

When a sex addict is so sick and tired of living a double life that they know they need to stop, they will disclose. Additionally, they are certain that telling their partner is the only way they can heal. Then they decide on a time and place to reveal the beginnings of the problems as well as the behaviours that led to their acting out. In order for it to qualify as disclosure, the addict's deliberate conviction to change, heal, or end the secretive lifestyle must be present.

However, the majority of sex addicts make what I refer to as a forced disclosure after being discovered. In actuality, forced disclosure never reveals the whole truth and is never really completely accurate. The betrayed partner is commonly stabilised and hushed with a forced disclosure while the full truth is still kept a secret to further impose deception. I usually advise the partners who have been betrayed to get ready for more because there will always be more.

Then there is the multiple disclosure, or as partners have called it, several stabbings or information dribbles. This happens more frequently when a sex addict keeps getting discovered or is gradually compelled to be honest because their partner is pressuring them or is discovering more. It might continue like this for a week, a month, a year, or until they take a polygraph.

Furthermore, I have never seen a sex addict fully disclose their addictive behaviours unless a polygraph test is imminent. Moreover, it is common practice, and I have grown accustomed to doing so, for me to wait until a few days or even a few minutes before the polygraph test before getting the full truth from the addicts.

The sex addict who is discovered will minimize, lie, answer only specific questions, blame, or shame the partner to escape their guilt and pain. The experience of being exposed to a partner's sex addiction is very different, intensifying and making both the information and the process of discovery traumatising. Even when betrayed partners have evidence of compulsive behaviour, it can still take a sex addict hours, days, or even months to come clean. A sex addict may periodically leave the house or refrain from communicating to their partners for days because they are unable to accept that they have been discovered while their partner has been traumatised by what they have discovered. Please keep in mind that your ability to heal as a betrayed partner depends on how you intentionally and with the help of a specialist address the discovery or disclosure of the betrayal. Typically, you are left with a lot of unanswered questions. The relationship, the sex addict, and their partner can all heal much more rapidly if the truth is out there rather than constantly carrying the shame and secrecy.

The discovery and disclosure frequently cause the betrayed partner to question not only the sincerity and integrity of their relationship but also the person they had assumed to be their intimate partner. In my research of intimate partners of sex addicts all betrayed partners questioned the true identity of their mates. One tearful woman expressed that she had been entirely unaware of her husband's true identity and stated:

> *Until I found out, in 2019, I never knew he had a problem. I didn't have a single idea before then. If you had asked me what I valued most about our relationship, I would have said his fidelity and loyalty. It was the furthest thing from my mind, and I never once questioned this.*

Others compared it to unwittingly sleeping with the enemy. All betrayed partners appeared to have obvious difficulties in identifying and engaging with their partner, as if he was someone else. They all worried whether the person they loved and trusted was who he claimed to be and whether he had ever loved them. One woman said:

'I started to think, Who am I married to?

I see the man I loved and married and [had] been with for more than 30 years, and I think of the things he has done, and it seems like two different people. I can't put the two together because that is a different person ... and I want that comfort, and I feel no comfort.'.

Betrayed partners frequently go through severe trauma following discovery or disclosure. They often experience trauma from betrayal that requires validation, support, and professional assistance. Unfortunately, because of the stigma attached to this particular addiction, the partners don't get the support they require and instead endure their suffering in silence.

My husband has always been my best friend. When I learned about his sex addiction and hidden life, which I was unaware of, we had been married for 20 years and had five children together. One evening when he was out, a message appeared on his iPad. He recently purchased an Apple Watch, which he had previously connected to his iPad. I saw a message from an escort giving him a quote for her services, and arranging their meeting for later that week. To say that I was shocked and felt like my world had suddenly collapsed would be an understatement. I'm not sure how I made it through and eventually put the kids to bed.

For the first time, I transformed into a detective on a quest and read all of his emails and other texts I could get my hands on. To find out when and how he was spending our money, I looked through our bank accounts. I kept finding new things as I dug deeper. At times, I was on the verge of collapsing from shaking. On his PC, I found pictures and movies. There were sextings, dating site communications, Instagram messaging, and Facebook messages. I couldn't believe my devoted, shy husband and loving father could have committed such heinous acts. Who was this man? I had no idea that the entrance to hell had just opened and that I hadn't even entered it. I fell to my knees from shock. Everything I believed to be true about my life and my marriage was destroyed that night. The trauma and the suffering were unbearable. A few days later, after I thought he had told me everything, I learned of additional lies. He wanted to answer all of my questions and was ashamed and remorseful for what he had done, but unable to tell the whole truth. I was repeatedly traumatised and left broken with each new piece of information. I was unable to eat, sleep, or watch over my children. Chaos reigned throughout. Every time I thought I had uncovered it all there were more. . I requested him to take a polygraph test after our therapist suggested it because I had gotten tired of his repeated disclosures. The awful reality was revealed at that point. There were even more shocking revelations, just when I believed there couldn't possibly be any information worse than the ones I already knew. He had engaged in unprotected sex with sex workers. Additionally, he had other sexual interactions with men. I frequently yelled at him and questioned why he married me. Why wasn't I enough?

My best friend, whom I confided in, blamed me for staying and became distant from me. I struggled to survive for months. I was given a diagnosis of post-traumatic stress disorder, and even though its effects have subsided, I nevertheless feel constantly on high alert and waiting for the next possible disaster. I'm not the same person I used to be. Although I stayed in my marriage, it has been a difficult path for me because I don't trust easily. Along the way, I developed a dependency on alcohol to numb my pain and experienced suicidal thoughts.

I had to educate myself about sex addiction and the reasons behind my husband's actions. I uncovered details about his early life that he had kept a secret. He had experienced trauma in his childhood and was unsure of how to handle his unpleasant emotions. At first, I was furious with both him and myself for failing to recognise this sooner. When he found a sex addiction specialist I reluctantly agreed to accompany him, and it marked the start of his recovery and our relationship restoration. Although the journey has not been smooth, we are moving forwards. Even when he is doing well, there have been numerous occasions when I have just wanted to die and end this nightmare. Nevertheless, the truth, in the words of my therapist, is "that what happened is your reality so let's deal with it because no matter how much you want to reverse it is impossible." In the past I kept asking why, but I've since discovered that in sex addiction, the answer may never be understood, so accepting that was crucial. Before I was able to forgive, we had to face a long and difficult journey through hell. I honestly hope that neither I nor our relationship will be defined by his addiction.

Whether you decide to leave or stay together as a couple, the journey is extremely difficult, but you can make it through and survive. Although it may seem unusual, I know that my husband considers me to be the love of his life and I am slowly accepting that I am his.

Jessica, wife of a sex addict

CHAPTER 5

Betrayal trauma caused by discovery and disclosure of sex addiction

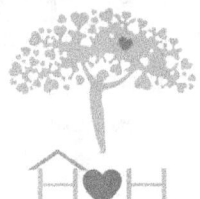

Discovery and/or disclosure of sex addiction= Betrayal Trauma or relational betrayal= PTSD

Jennifer Freyd, a psychologist, developed the idea of betrayal trauma for the first time in 1991. She identified it as a particular trauma that occurs in significant social interactions where the betrayed person has to keep up a relationship with the betrayer for support or safety. According to the betrayal trauma theory, damage to attachment bonds, such as those between a parent and child or romantic partners, can result in long-lasting trauma.

When someone we depend on for survival or who we have a strong emotional attachment to significantly breaks our trust, it can cause betrayal trauma. Knowing about the sex addiction or partner's secrets is particularly traumatising due to the past lies the betrayed partner has believed. Excruciating pain, anxiety, and shame result when a loved one violates the relational integrity. The question often asked is - *Why did I allow myself to be so fooled?*

Regardless of how the information was acquired, finding that a partner has a sex addiction can be heartbreaking and traumatic. It can be a life changing moment and feel like the ultimate betrayal. Like other traumatic occurrences, the intensity of the moment might be kept inside. As a result, the betrayed partner can experience symptoms that are similar to those experienced by war veterans and victims of crime. These individuals generally present with PTSD responses and are hypervigilant and in a survival mood because they don't perceive their environment or world safe anymore.

When there is betrayal in a relationship, the attachment bond is shattered, and the trauma of the betrayal renders the relationship a threat rather than a haven for emotional safety.

Betrayal Trauma is a serious psychological wound. When such a wound arises as a result of a discovering or disclosing compulsive sexual behaviours of a partner, the brain of the betrayed reacts by activating the limbic system, which is the survival component of the brain. All rationality is lost when the limbic system takes over. The prefrontal cortex, the rational portion of the brain, shuts off while the limbic system—which is hardwired for survival—is active. The sufferer receives a signal from their limbic system that

Betrayal trauma caused by discovery and disclosure of sex addiction

their life is in danger. The fight, flight, freeze, or fawn response will consequently be triggered.

Traumatic betrayal is the experience of being wronged by the deliberate actions or omissions of a trusted person. Disclosure of private information without consent, untrustworthiness, cheating, and deception are the most frequent types of betrayal. They might cause a great deal of suffering and be distressing. The aftermath of a betrayal might involve shock, grief and loss, pathological obsession, diminished self-esteem and self-trust, and rage. These symptoms often bring about life-altering changes. The betrayer frequently serves as a permanent trauma trigger, and betrayal can alter the mind and thought.

Betrayal Trauma most frequently results from:

- Physical, sexual, and emotional abuse of children, including coercion, gaslighting, verbal abuse.
- Discovery or disclosure of partner's betrayal, including emotional, physical, sexual, financial and spiritual betrayal.

Betrayed trauma is distinguished considerably from other types of trauma by the experience of being betrayed by a significant relationship, such as a parent, caregiver, or an intimate partner who is relied upon for care, safety and assistance.

Because the victim relies on the offender to meet their physiological, social, psychological, and/or emotional needs, they frequently are compelled to alter their attitude to maintain the relationship.

As a result, a betrayed partner could experience:

- **Cognitive dissonance** -the capacity to hold two opposing ideas simultaneously, minimisation and downplaying the seriousness of sex addict's actions.
- **Betrayal blindness** -inability to recognise betrayal despite abundant proof. By avoiding what is too unpleasant or terrifying to face, this type of psychological blindness serves as a coping mechanism to ensure their mental and emotional well-being.

As part of my job, I frequently encounter the partners of sex addicts who attend therapy for what they incorrectly think are issues in communications or in the relationship. After learning about the real issues, some partners use denial, minimisation, or betrayal blindness to draw attention away from their sex addict partner. I've seen sex addicts talk about some of their problematic actions and choices, only to have their partners brush them off as normal and tell them they don't want to hear any more because they don't think those issues are significant. When I encounter this kind of individual, I choose not to work with the couple and instead extend an invitation for them to return once they have both acknowledged their real concerns and are committed to resolve them as a united team.

The imposed trauma, suffering and grief experienced by some betrayed partners are only made worse by the addict's criminal activity, rejection and exclusions from organisations, arrest, and impending punishment. There are challenges including the fear of exposure and loneliness, financial difficulties, or social embarrassment. In some extreme but not uncommon cases, the addict even had a totally different family, children, and financial commitments.

The brain retains extremely accurate notes of every aspect of the experience following trauma. The brain stores all of this information,

Betrayal trauma caused by discovery and disclosure of sex addiction

which is available at the slightest trigger. Because of this, a betrayed partner may occasionally react to circumstances that may appear unconnected to the original trauma.

For example, seeing a woman on the street who resembles a woman the sex addict acted out with, hearing a song, seeing a couple who can serve as a reminder of a loving relationship, seeing billboards with sexual imagery, watching a movie, looking at old family photos, being in places where specific memories of times the sex addict was lying have been revealed, being in places linked to the discovery or disclosure of the betrayals, time periods linked to past betrayals, and anniversaries or other special celebratory occasions- all of these circumstances and more have the potential to trigger trauma reactions.

Once the betrayed partner's trauma brain is activated, her entire body and mind are then hijacked, and all of her attention is directed towards surviving the attack or assault, which her physicality and emotionality experience as ground hog day. This simplified insight explains why betrayed partners frequently exhibit sudden over-reacting or seemingly irrational, erratic, or even misinterpreted as crazy reactions.

The experience of one betrayed partner was as follows:

> *When I would lose my mind completely over what seemed to be a minor indiscretion committed by my partner, a somewhat unremarkable occurrence, or a pointless incident, I used to feel guilty and embarrassed. Even I couldn't understand what I was doing. What was the matter with me? Why was I behaving in this odd way? Am I crazy? Will I ever get better and return to normal? I re-traumatize myself because I didn't know or understood that I was simply traumatised and that*

my behaviour was a reflection of my trauma symptoms. I felt normal once I realised that I had PTSD-related betrayal trauma, which improved my capacity for self-compassion. The most difficult aspect was that my husband didn't know how to assist me; instead, he would act angry, defensive, or simply dismissive. Naturally, my dysregulation would increase as a result of his response, and I would become more explosive every time. We both gradually gained knowledge of betrayal trauma and triggers. He developed active listening skills and empathy while supporting me, which really aided me and lessened my trauma symptoms till I was able to help myself more and more. We both now understand that for the trauma brain to deactivate, it requires empathy, validation, and compassion.

Kate, partner of a sex addict

In my recent research I found that 100% of intimate partners of sex addicts experienced PTSD symptoms upon discovery or disclosure of such behaviours. Each relapse that follows could exacerbate these symptoms in the future.

Trauma results in a loss in mental health when the betrayed partner is unable to sleep at night. Physical discomfort and crippling migraines can be brought on by emotional anxiety. Likewise, they may find it challenging to focus due to their anxious thoughts or panic attacks.

The memories, flashbacks and intrusive images recur in the mind. Perhaps they can remember a time when their sex addict partner made them feel unjustifiably guilty. Alternately, when they anticipated a problem but chose to dismiss it and disregard their own intuitions. And to make matters worse, they remember challenging their partner and being accused as crazy. As they begin to question everything about their relationship, even their fondest memories can seem like a significant deception or fake. On the other hand,

Betrayal trauma caused by discovery and disclosure of sex addiction

some betrayed partners can think they are unworthy of love or that they can't trust themselves. These people become trapped in false guilt and self-condemnation, and they begin to believe that they are flawed because of what has happened to them. They are once more going through a perfectly normal response to a betrayal of trust brought on by betrayal trauma.

How can betrayal trauma manifest itself?

Trauma is subjective, and its manifestations depend entirely on the individual, how their brain perceives the threat they face, and their past experiences. An illustration of what a betrayed trauma present itself is as follows:

My trauma was completely in control of me and would frequently swing between extremes.. In order to avoid the anguish of being awake and having to confront my life's reality, I would sleep for hours every day. However, I was unable to sleep at night because of constant nightmares that reproduced my husband's compulsive sexual behaviours with others.

I experienced a period of fixation and obsession with self-harm behaviours and suicidal ideas. I always felt confused or fuzzy, as if my brain was having trouble processing or connecting information. Simple, everyday tasks all of a sudden seemed complex and challenging to do. The anguish of this manner of existence shocked me. At first, I was completely unable to manage my emotions. I had a tendency to react strongly to even the smallest problems. There was an undercurrent of fear and panic underneath everything I did, felt, said, or perceived. I had the impression that I was always sobbing uncontrollably while barely keeping myself from collapsing. I had no idea that someone could go through this much pain and still survive. My anger was roaring. I used to occasionally be afraid of my own thoughts and my ability to hurt my partner. On one occasion, when I was slicing vegetables, my husband simply approached me and asked if I needed help. If I hadn't controlled myself at that point, I probably would have committed murder or serious bodily harm. When we tried to discuss at night after the kids were in bed, it typically ended in a meltdown, shouting, and terrible verbal fights when real revelations would seep out, which continued to happen for what felt like an eternity. I was inconsolable, kicking, screaming, swinging my fists, sobbing, and feeling drained. The anger had become a potent narcotic on my body, and I appeared to be dependent on it. It initially gave me a temporary break from the crushing sense of worthlessness and defeat that I was experiencing most of the time. In my chaotic life, anger gave me a way to express my excruciating pain and a way to make my husband experience some suffering. However, the brief relief was quickly followed by remorse, shame, guilt, and additional pain. Having experienced trauma, I was persuaded that I was completely useless and that my husband was for ever damage goods. To reconnect and learn how to control my rage and pain, both of us needed intensive counselling, which we have been receiving for three years this year.

Anne, wife of a sex addict

Healing is possible, whether you choose to continue being a couple or want to go your separate ways. You are deserving of compassion during this trying period in your life. Don't put off finding happiness until everything in life is ideal. Unless you make your own happiness and fulfilment because you are capable of doing it and because you deserve it, there is practically never the ideal moment in life. Ultimately, many betrayed partners will simply call it quits rather than put themselves through what could end up being quite a battle. The reality is needing to deal with the highs and lows of the recovery process with the potential for occasional relapses. Therefore, during

Betrayal trauma caused by discovery and disclosure of sex addiction

the ongoing process of recovering from sex addiction, the betrayed partners who have decided to remain in their relationships must be realistic and aware of the considerable possibility of further intentional or unintentional re-traumatization instances.

The following requirements must be met by betrayed partners who decide to continue their relationship with a recovered sex addict:

1) Commit themselves to recovering from the betrayal trauma.
2) Participate in and support their partner's effective sex addiction recovery.
3) Work collectively to restore the relationship.
4) Be willing to work on their own self-development.

CHAPTER 6

The multifaceted effects of betrayal trauma

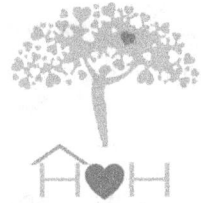

The emotional impacts of betrayal trauma- The sufferers resiliency: Your level of resilience as well as the coping and self-protective techniques you currently use in daily life can have a significant impact on how psychologically devastating a sex addiction betrayal is for you. Your mental health may be seriously impacted by SA-related infidelity, including but not limited to body image issues, diminished sexual confidence, and low self-esteem.

Self-blame/ false guilt: Infidelity associated to SA frequently has a self-blame aftereffect. Trauma frequently leads betrayed partners to doubt and self-loath.

In my study, 66% of betrayed partners blamed themselves and felt responsible for their partner's SA. They all had feelings like:

- *What is wrong with me?*
- *Did I cause my partner's SA?*
- *Maybe I am not good enough?*
- *Should I have given him more intimacy, attention or sex?*
- *I'm not emotionally fulfilling him, so he needs to go somewhere else.*
- *All of this happened after I had children. In my head, I still have to make sure it isn't my fault, and he made choices. I would ruminate and have quite a bit of anger towards myself for not seeing this ... It took me a while to realise that quite a bit of the anger I felt was towards myself for not seeing this ... Then I began to wonder what was going on for me, that I didn't notice. All my fault! Not enough sex, he was lonely, if I had sex with him more often, he would never have looked! This haunted me for months.*

Since you cannot change the past, keep your attention on the here and now, and if you find yourself blaming yourself for the betrayal, acknowledge it, practise self-compassion, and give yourself permission to stop. You can avoid and control this psychological impact of betrayal trauma by simply shifting your inner dialogue to a more empowering and loving one, such as *I am enough, valued, and worthy of love and respect*.

Panic attacks and anxiety: Since your entire existence has been turned upside down, the pain of betrayal is likely to have a profound psychological impact, including panic attacks and/or anxious feelings. Several betrayed partners have reported of these negative consequences:

The multifaceted effects of betrayal trauma

Since learning of my husband's SA, I have suffered from severe panic attacks and social anxiety. During these attacks, my heart would beat, my chest would feel tight and achy, I would get a lump in my throat, and my jaw would hurt. If I do not experience a panic attack, I will be waiting for one to occur.

Tanya, wife of a sex addict

Your panic attacks and degree of anxiety are understandable given the level of trauma you have experienced and you might think about getting a medical evaluation. Some useful skills to use following trauma management therapy include deep breathing exercises, meditation, self-care routines, walking, swimming, drawing, listening to music, and learning self-regulation techniques.

Diminished self-esteem: When you are in a relationship with a sex addict, it will be tough to reconcile the fact that the person you loved, trusted, and invested your life in has betrayed you by engaging in sexual or emotional intimacy with another. You'll start to question why you weren't chosen instead of others who were taller, smaller, better looking, slimmer, or who catered to your partner's every desire.

One betrayed partner gave the following account of her lowered self-esteem:

I felt unworthy shortly after finding out about his infidelity and SA, and as a result, I no longer had any self-esteem. We had established this partnership and our way of life together, so even though I often felt like leaving, I stayed. I've included time, both of our youths, as well as the fact that we had a child. I don't want my child to have to deal with having divorced parents. I hold out hope that I may someday recover my self-esteem and stop negatively comparing myself to others. It is agony to move around with low self-esteem and listening to the voice in my head that shouts that I am not attractive, skinny enough, or good enough.

Jasmine, partner of a sex addict

Physical impacts of betrayal trauma- Short-term stress is easier for human beings to handle than persistent, long-lasting stress (i.e., betrayal trauma). Trauma overload occurs when the mind and body are unable to unwind, leading to increased and ongoing anxiety and trepidation. This can reduce coping mechanisms, lead to mental exhaustion, and result in a variety of physical illnesses. As was already established, physical symptoms might involve a variety of problems, including body image, weight loss or gain, sleep problems, rage outbursts, nausea, intolerance to close contact, sobbing and screaming episodes, fainting, hair loss, and more. Bessel van der Kolk elaborates on how trauma can have substantial physiological effects on the brain and body in his book The Body Keeps the Score. The body recalls the trauma of betrayal, whereas the brain may block it out. This may show up as throat infections, migraines, digestive problems, persistent exhaustion, overeating, bowel distress and sleep problems.

Initially feeling dejected, betrayed partners frequently develop several physical illnesses, heightened vigilance in an effort to ascertain what their sex addict partners' true motivations are. They frequently make control attempts or take detective roles. Betrayed partners may have a flood of fears and feelings about their partner and relationship as a result of the trauma of betrayal. They can doubt the sincerity of the relational bond. They could wonder how their partner was able to carry out such a serious act of betrayal. They constantly ponder whether their relationship and their personal health would ever feel normal again. Whether the sufferer realised that their partner had betrayed them repeatedly or only once, the effects of the betrayal

The multifaceted effects of betrayal trauma

trauma can have complex negative effects that can continue to give for a long time post discovery or disclosure.

A defining characteristic of betrayal trauma that is commonly present is intrusive thoughts about the betrayal. As a result, the betrayed partner could become fixated on searching for indicators of ongoing deception. They frequently begin by searching their partner's phone records, bank account information, and internet browsing history.

The primary cause of partner betrayal trauma is the way the significant other (sex addict) utterly disregards all of their partner's shared thoughts and emotions when they engage in compulsive behaviours with themselves or others. They disregard the integrity, values, thoughts, emotions, and priorities of their partner. They intentionally neglect the priceless privilege of being with them. The partner gave their heart to the sex addict before this relationship even began, not realising how it would be broken and stomped upon.

The betrayed partner discussed their aspirations, triumphs, goals, dreams, hardships, and fears. They shared their hopes for the kids and the future. They arrived at the right time to offer the sex addict encouragement. They sometimes even showed their partners enormous affection while ignoring their major shortcomings.

Nevertheless, the sex addict, makes the decision to betray them with the invisible mistress (SA) or through porn, and infidelity. The sex addict's behavioural message to the betrayed partner is: *Your heart has little to no significance to me, thus I choose myself and what my heart desire while deciding to forsake and reject your heart*. All these negative experiences can take a toll on the hurt partner's physical health.

According to one betrayed partner who took part in my study, her physical effects were as follows:

In just three weeks, I dropped 10 kg. I started to have an eating disorder and had trouble sleeping. Prior to beginning therapy, I briefly experienced depression and developed a shopping addiction. Still today I don't get out much, and I've given up my job permanently because I can't take the stress. I learned that he had given me a STI and that I had grown ill with an auto immune disease. Both chronic headaches and intermittent depression are still issues for me.

Janette, partner of a sex addict

Spiritual impacts of betrayal trauma- Another consequence of betrayal trauma experienced by hurt partners is spiritual crises or perplexity. The broad concept of spirituality encompasses a connection to God or a higher power, as well as a sense of mystery and wonder about one's own experiences. It might be claimed that spirituality is unique, unique to each person, and in many ways, indefinable as the spot where humanity and the Divine meet.

Additionally, spirituality is fundamentally about living human experience and is inherently geared towards discovery and connection to god or other higher power.

All relationships with our significant other, partner and other people are shaped by our spirituality, whether or not we identify as religious or spiritual. We all engage in some form of spiritual practise and possess particular beliefs. Our spirits and these ideas profoundly influence who we are. They also set our moral standards and enable us to exist outside of ourselves yet connecting to a designer or higher power.

Sex addiction and betrayal trauma can have an equal impact on people of all ages and religious backgrounds. These conditions are not exclusive to any one practise, spirituality or belief. Spirituality

The multifaceted effects of betrayal trauma

is the very real interior element of ourselves that connects us to God or a Higher Power and genuinely influences all our relationships. In actuality, our spirit frequently becomes aware of problems in a relationship before we do.

Serious spiritual repercussions for the betrayed partner result from the sex addict's disrespect for their partner's spiritual beliefs and spirit. Occasionally, this reality may bring them much more agony than they could ever experience physically since spirituality penetrates the souls so profoundly. It is also challenging to accept because everyone's relationships and way of life are so based on their beliefs.

In my research, I found that the betrayed partners suffered severe spiritual repercussions regardless of their level of spirituality or religiosity. For 83% of betrayed partners who believed in a god entity or a higher power they initially felt disconnected and started by questioning the fairness in allowing the betrayal to occur, contributing to their initial disconnection from their faith or spirituality. This situation was more challenging when sufferers of faith attempted to seek refuge in their faith-based communities only to be advised to forgive their partner or that the betrayal was not serious. This meant that the betrayed perceived their experiences and grief to be minimised or even invalidated. For some hurt partners, the lack of support from the church or other faith based communities was an indicator of a lack of support from God. Without actual validation for the betrayed partners' experiences, holding the offender accountable, or enforcing consequences, those communities seemingly overlooked or minimised the betrayal. Furthermore, the absence of validation signified that the sex addicts had God's approval and betrayed partners perceived their sex addict mates as extensions of God, perpetuating the patriarchy. While the sex addicts had kept their partners in the dark by maintaining secrets and acting deceptively, in their eyes, God/higher power had done the same, by failing to reveal the offences, and was therefore an accomplice in the deception. Several hurt partners spiritual crises were centred on their broader perception of their spirituality. Consequently, many betrayed partners' spiritual underpinnings became unstable, if not impaired. In this space, they withdrew spiritually and could not confide in others or rely on their spiritual power, exacerbating their isolation, stigmatisation and loneliness.

One betrayed partner described her spiritual challenges as follow:

At the start, I didn't understand why this would happen to someone like me who had been strong, spiritual and a dedicated member of my church community. Since I remember, I have been actively involved in the church. My family has a history of serving as missionaries and pastors. For us, church simply represented a way of life. But it was too tense for me to take my eyes off the dreadfully traumatic reality I shared with my husband for a moment to turn to God for assistance. I frequently cried out, "Why?" What caused it, and why? Why did you allow this to happen to me? I was brought up in a very strong spiritual home and Christian family, so why did I have to endure such suffering? Although I am not perfect, I believe I have always been faithful to God and have never strayed from His path by engaging in risky or rebellious teenage behaviour. I wonder why He did not protect me for my loyalty but punished me instead?

And perhaps, like Job in the Bible account, everything was suddenly stolen from him despite him being a devoted servant. Why did I get that treatment. Now, I have no faith and don't believe anything at all. Having a God with a plan and all that is now, in my opinion, nonsense. Now that I think about it, I wonder why a loving God, if there is one, would not have

The multifaceted effects of betrayal trauma

allowed me to find out sooner. Why? There were several chances for me to learn more. Since no good God would ever treat another being in such a cruel and spiteful manner, I believe he is either a very evil or vengeful god. Even my worst enemy wouldn't be the target of this.

Bianca, partner of a sex addict

Social and relational impacts of betrayal trauma- Loss of the relationship you thought you had: your marriage or relationship, at least as you viewed it before, doesn't actually exist anymore. Whether you stay in the relationship or break it off, your life will never be the same again. You might be able to start over and construct another relationship that is just as precious as the one you thought you had, but you can never replace what you previously had. You don't have much control over the profound psychological agony brought on by betrayal trauma. You need to give yourself some space to mourn since you have truly lost something. Create time and space for yourself, allow yourself to lament and to vent your anger, agony, anxiety, and guilt. Spend some time alone so that you can properly process the loss. Gradually, as you do intentional work to heal you will learn to create a new normal and re-integrate your life . Most betrayed partners in my recent study found themselves unable to maintain some relationships due to blame being transferred onto them, being criticised by others for continuing their relationships or being criticised for choosing to separate. One hurt partner commented:

I feel so embarrassed. Until I found out the truth, I never knew there was a major problem. I didn't have a single idea before then. If you had asked me what I valued most about our relationship, I would have said his fidelity and loyalty. It was the furthest thing from my mind, and I never once questioned this. Afterwards, I was afraid that my family and friends would judge my decision to stay in my marriage. My family would almost certainly have pushed me to leave him. His SA has destroyed a lot of my relationships. I have lost my best friend because she couldn't understand why I would stay. Although, my parents and siblings don't know the whole truth about him, they don't want to hear about it either. We've all broken up and I have been forced to withdraw from everyone, I'm so ashamed.

Janice, partner of a sex addict

The betrayed partners might also grow distrustful of everyone, but especially of men. Others seem to vanish into a life of going through the motions and total numbness. They live by filling their time with activities that prevent them from having time to feel their feelings. They lose any ability to feel anything, whether it be painful or pleasurable.

My same research found that due to a common lack of truthful disclosure and ongoing deception from the sex addicts the betrayed partners are compelled to do detective work to uncover the truth. However, once they uncover more facts, it seems that the veil has been removed, and they will now continue their truth-seeking on their own terms until a coherent story can be constructed to address the what, why and how. This process involves a great deal of anticipation of heartache and trauma, which is made even worse when further truth is discovered through their detective work rather than voluntary disclosure. For betrayed partners, this stage of going on the hunt resembles hell, more betrayal, and causes constant hypervigilance and re-traumatisation.

The experience of one betrayed partner participant in my study conducting detective work to uncover the truth is best illustrated by the following:

The multifaceted effects of betrayal trauma

In my quest and hunt for the truth, I examined every single piece of paper I came across to see whether it had a password or a link to something. I found that my husband had a completely different name, email, and other things set up under a phoney name. So, every time I learned something new about his other life, it was disturbing. It probably took me close to three months to find out more about him, although at the time it seemed to go on forever. I wished I could wake up because it seemed like I was in a nightmare. He proceeded to downplay and dismiss any problems he could have throughout this period. He pretended to still be the horny guy who had gotten a little out of hand. But at this time, I had discovered hotel invoices, proof of more than 247 women, and I had used Google Maps to follow every single journey he had taken for the past few months. It became increasingly difficult for him to maintain that nothing was wrong because thanks to my detective work, I had spreadsheets documenting what he did. Even though I was poor with computers he was still trying to gaslight me and manipulate me. During that time period I would be really upset and call him repeatedly at work, check his phone, get on his computer, and search through it. I just felt crazy and so out of control because how can I know if I don't spy or control him? I needed him to tell me the truth, but he wasn't able so how can I ever trust him, myself or others again?

Hanna, partner of a sex addict

Figure 3 depicts what the betrayed partner goes through after the initial discovery or disclosure of their sex addict partners.

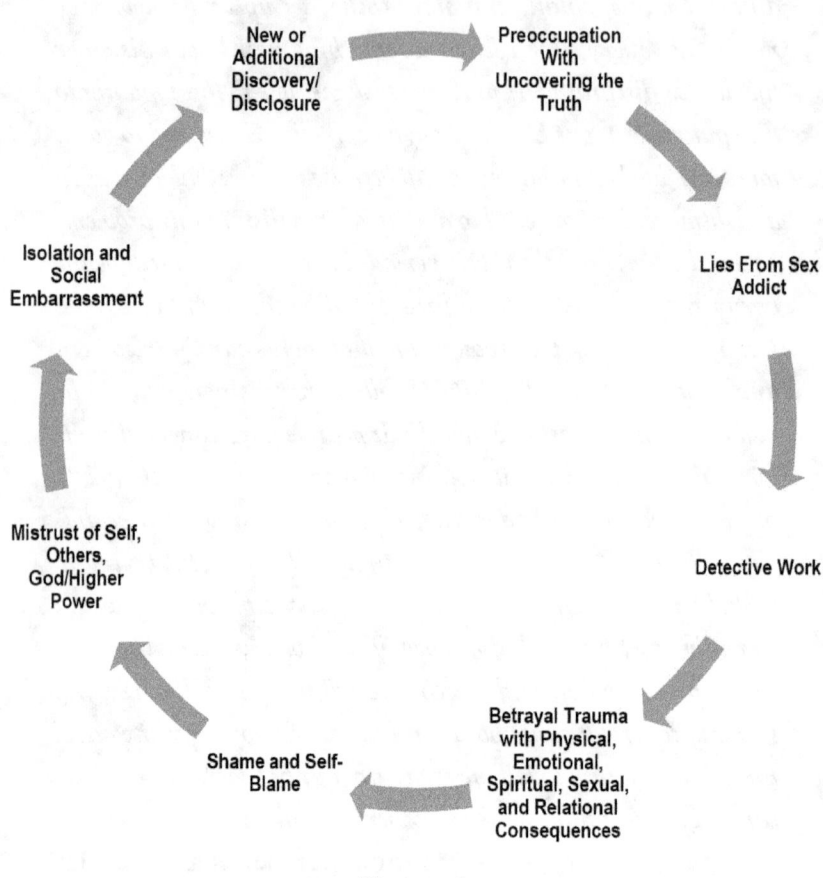

Figure 3

A partner may feel alone and isolated after being betrayed. A betrayed partner could feel ambivalent, fearful, ashamed or stigmatised by the lack of knowledge about SA, about asking for help or even knowing how to ask for help.

For a variety of reasons, individuals might not want their family and friends to know what they are going through. They could feel

The multifaceted effects of betrayal trauma

some sort of personal responsibility for the betrayal or even feel compelled to uphold their partner's reputation. Particularly if the person has experienced early adverse life experiences or has been violated, their trauma may be reactivated, which can then worsen their trauma symptoms with potentially life-altering consequences. When dealing with a terrible situation within a relationship that is so important, it can be difficult to know what to do. The romantic partnership is a social unit. Individuals may make the journey together, participate in the same activities and events, and go out in public together as a couple. The social betrayal component of partner betrayal trauma results from the fact that sufferers start to wonder how people view both of them as a result of the betrayal.

On an internal and outward level, there is social deception. From an internal standpoint, many partners frequently have this nagging feeling of doubting whether others are aware of what is actually happening. When such individuals come across individuals in the street, they may wonder: *Do they know? Did they know then? What do they think about what happened? How do they see me?*

The betrayed partner's perception of how others view them, own self-worth, self-efficacy, lovability, and right to exist all suffer as a result of the cognitive distortions generated in the wake of trauma. These distortions typically centre on oneself rather than the outside world or other people. Trauma distorts even the most fundamental self-perceptions, beliefs and meaning making processes.

Numerous factors, such as the duration of the relationship with the sex addict and how well the victim thought they knew them, affect the relational and social aspects of betrayal trauma. The social or interpersonal impacts of betrayal appear to look like avoidance behaviours from a distance. The hurt partner refrains from engaging in certain activities, applies self-imposed isolation, avoids visiting specific places or social gatherings, or meeting specific individuals since doing so forces them to reflect on what happened. This is to escape encounters with people who might find out about the betrayal, because the suffers frequently project their internal feelings onto the outside environment. As a result of the betrayal, the relational and social structures are significantly disrupted, and the betrayed partner's fear about their social environment grows.

It's special and significant to note how the betrayed partner is coping with the trauma. They might put on weight if they try to eat their way out of discomfort. They might become too cautious, hyper vigilant and overly concerned about safety if this is the case. If they try to exert control, they could develop OCD and find themselves compulsively fixated on everything. The betrayal ultimately affects them on every level of their being.

The effects of trauma caused by betrayal on the physical and mental well-being of the betrayed partner are outlined in the list below, which is not all-inclusive:

- A sense of being enveloped in a "haze" (dissociation).
- Feelings of helplessness or despair, panic and disbelief.
- Jaw clenching.
- Avoiding social interactions.
- Denial or avoiding acknowledging the trueness of what has happened.
- Experiencing depression, lack of concentration, worthlessness, self-doubt, self-loathing, body image issues.
- Obsessive thoughts about their sex addict partner.
- Overeating or under eating.

The multifaceted effects of betrayal trauma

- Excessive screen time.
- Compulsive shopping.
- Excessive drinking.
- Panic attacks, poor sleep, flashbacks.
- Nightmares.
- Anger outbursts.
- Fearfulness.
- Shame and guilt.
- Social embarrassment and shame.
- Headaches, developing autoimmune illnesses.
- Lack of emotional regulation.
- Sexual dysfunction (inability to enjoy sexual intimacy with sex addict partner, loss of sexual freedom or hypersexuality).
- Constant triggers about the experiences.
- Crying.
- Developing physical illnesses.
- Lack of decision making.
- Lack of self-trust and self-esteem.
- Feeling unattractive.
- Inability to fulfill daily tasks.
- Self-harm behaviours and suicidal thoughts.
- Losing faith in God/Higher power.
- Bleak outlook on life and future.

Sexual impacts of betrayal trauma

Sexual intimacy is thought to be the most sacred interaction between two individuals. It means exposing your complete vulnerability and giving your full self to your partner or significant other. In my study I found one of the most powerful and pervasive effects of betrayal trauma, is how it affects the hurt partner's sexuality. I found that the effects include diminished sexual desire, feelings of unworthiness, sexual ambiguity/uncertainty, loss of sexual freedom and pleasure, sexual shutting down, aversion to touch, fear, and anxiety—all of which have been compared to the effects of sexual trauma or rape on victims in other studies. As well as issues with body image, difficulty getting aroused, or feeling emotionally numb during sexual activity.

The adverse sexual impacts also impinged on the female partners' relational sexual satisfaction. Lack of sexual freedom meant having involuntary and disquieting mental images of the partner watching pornography or engaging sexually with others and the inability to erase these mental triggers during sexual intimacy.

Sexual intimacy is frequently seen as sacred, and sex addiction dangerously transgresses this sacredness through severe boundary violations. Some betrayed partners may experience hysterical hypersexuality or trauma bonding states, especially in the early stages of discovery or disclosure and due to shock. They crave more sex, engage in more imaginative sexual experimentation, and have greater verbal interaction during sex in this phase. In my study I found that 75% or betrayed partners participated in transient hysterical hypersexuality with their sex addict partner shortly after revelations. For the hurt partner, engaging in transitory hypersexual behaviours constituted a form of trauma bonding that appeared to signify re-attachment and a form of out-competing individuals with whom their male partner had engaged sexually, or of out-competing intrusive sexual images. Engaging in hypersexual activities seemingly meant feeling good enough or, in some cases, gratifying their partner's sexual demands to prevent them from seeking external sexual pleasure. Hypersexuality with the sex addict partner as a form of trauma bonding resulted from trauma conflict or trauma response, which triggered trauma connections in those cases. However, these transient behaviours tended to cause re-traumatisation due to the subsequent shame and embarrassment. Others could experience a void inside. They either feel paralysed and no longer desire sex with the sex addict partner or are repulsed by the thought of it.

The loss of faith in the sacred source of sexuality in their relationship is the root of these trauma responses. According to a participant in my study the betrayal trauma impacts on her sexuality were as follows:

> *I constantly feel on edge and like, do you just want to do this because of porn? I thought we had to renew our sexual connection, and tried to have as much sex as possible with him but it never worked... There was a period where I became a little more hypersexual, and that's when I started feeling like a pincushion. All that hypersexuality re-traumatised me more and gave me more shame. I still find it quite difficult to maintain sexual intimacy. Although it is improving, I would be lying if I said it hasn't been tough. I get endless triggers when I see him, I have to keep my eyes closed during sex. Even after so many years of recovery, I remain permanently broken.*
>
> **Laura, partner of a sex addict**

Impact of betrayal trauma on the outlook of life and future

My research revealed that the outlook on life and future of betrayal trauma has a significant impact. I found that betrayed partners are often apprehensive about each new day and what the future might hold. Healing is a multidimensional, slow, nonlinear process that is unique for each individual and may remain incomplete for an extended period of time for most of them due to the uncertainty of future. Living in this state of uncertainty means the betrayed partners have to give up most of their life plans and dreams, as those visions can no longer coexist with the realities of their lives. Uncertainty is the result of a person encountering unpredictable outcomes of an event, resulting in feelings of self-doubt and a state of not knowing.

Dread of the unknown is a fundamental fear of human beings contributing to negative emotions. According to Hall (2016), betrayed partners frequently face considerable doubts, worries, and uncertainties, whether they remain in or leave their partnerships. For most betrayed partners, the future is changed, as it is no longer based on a firm foundation of their partnership, which harms their outlook on life.

My research also showed that betrayed partners lose faith in both their current and potential future partners, which has a negative impact on their worldview. Similar to how they feel and think about themselves, others, and their future, such people have a negative self-view. These unfavourable feelings and ideas may act as a barrier against potential suffering in the future, but they have the potential to turn into shackles over time.

Additionally, an uncertain outlook on life, and engaging in unpleasant thoughts and feelings seems to be a type of protection against or preparation for future harm. Holding onto and preparing for such ideas and feelings, however, also can lead to preoccupations and increased suffering. Furthermore, for some betrayed partners uncertainty of future prospects may include financial concerns and uncertainties.

CHAPTER 7

Betrayal trauma shatters the most significant aspect of the relationship - relational trust

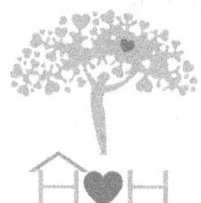

We are all driven to need some form of attachment simply to survive. We need to know the person with whom we share this primary attachment—this trust—is there for us. We need to know that we matter to them.

For most adults, this secure attachment is found in our mates the ones committed to us. The ones who vowed to be there for us in sickness and in health, for richer or poorer, for better and for worse. They promised to be available and connected to us. They promised to put us first in their life, forsaking all others.

Betrayal by the mates who made those vows reveals an ugly reality about our trust:

- I wasn't first in your life.
- I didn't matter.
- You're not there for me.
- You can't be trusted.

When the one who vowed to be our secure attachment deceives us and chooses someone (or something) else instead of us, what happens to that deep trust we depended on? What happens to that attachment? What do we do?

If the unfaithful spouse seems unwilling to make the necessary efforts to right the wrong and work at minimizing future violations, then the hurt spouse will find little incentive to attempt reconciliation and restore trust. Trust and forgiveness are not the same. You can forgive someone but still not consider him or her safe enough to trust. In the case of infidelity, before you trust, you need to know that you matter to them, that they will be responsive to you, and that they want to be there for you. Without these conditions in place, there is little on which to base trust. Before you willingly move toward a reconciliation of hearts, you want to know that the person who broke their commitment to you is safe. You need to see your mate actively taking the steps necessary to restore trust and safety.

After being betrayed, it severely affects your ability to trust, which is normal. Trauma brought on by betrayal might occasionally mirror the lingering, sharp pain experienced after being suddenly kicked in the face. I compare the betrayal of sex addiction to deliberately and repeatedly driving over the partner with a heavy truck. The challenging aspect is that the perpetrator is not a complete stranger. Rather, it's a person you adore and never in a million years would have imagined would behave in such a manner. It becomes difficult to put your trust in them again. Ultimately, it may be challenging to trust anyone once more.

Living in such a reality can be extremely challenging and toxic, even though it might take a lifetime to adjust to the effects of such a breach and you have every right to be suspicious and not trust and make the offender pay for the harm they have inflicted.

Trust is a mental and emotional act. It is a situation where you emotionally open up to others while also trusting that they have your best interests at heart and won't exploit you. It makes sense that this is the case when you have evaluated the probability of costs and benefits and come to the conclusion that the individual will act predictably.

Your heart must heal, and enough time must pass before you can rationally determine that the person who betrayed you is now trustworthy. Only then can trust be re-established. Give yourself time and space to heal up till you get to the point where you can say this. Be patient.

You might not be able to predict whether your partner will once again deceive you or relapse. To love an imperfect person is, in all honesty, to take a chance. There are no risk-free relationships unless you bury yourself deep in the ground and barricade everyone from seeing or touching your heart. You don't want to let fear rule your life. Never let fear rule your thoughts; always keep life in mind. If you're ever going to trust someone, you're going to have to concede that the prospect of being hurt exists. However, if you can believe that your partner has a willing heart and it's not their intention to hurt you, you can at least take a chance. Have faith in your improved ability to spot dishonesty. You are not the same naïve individual who was in the past deceived and kept in the dark. You are a brand-new creature with razor-sharp radars that can spot deception miles away. While before you couldn't recognise the one who was living with you, I'll bet that now you can walk down the street and easily spot the sex addicts. Yes, you don't know what you don't know. But once you know what you know, you can't unknow it.

Vaughan (2003) argues in her book The Monogamy Myth that relying on the idea of marriage and presuming people will be devoted to one another endangers relationships.

Safety is more crucial to a secure romantic relationship than trust. Trust can be replaced with lots of open and honest dialogue if partners have a safe place to talk. Some betrayed partners assume their relationship is over and doomed simply because they lost their initial trust in their partner. However, an emphasis on safety provides a practical roadmap for couples to reconnect. Recognize that although it could take some time, initially, you don't require trust to succeed in your relationship post discovery or disclosure, you need safety. Therefore, look for safety in your sex addict's behaviour and language. Additionally, concentrate on building a safe partnership through finding creative ways to express your worries and fears.

Find other couples or individuals who are overcoming a circumstance like yours and take note of their failures and achievements. In the beginning of your journey, value safety first and trust will develop.

Acknowledge that you need to take the necessary actions to help ensure the safety of yourself, your partner, and your family by getting the adequate support immediately. Give up expecting life to be fair; stop pondering why this isn't the case; and just accept things as they are. Your suffering and grief will only grow as a result of such unreasonable expectations.

I always tell the betrayed partners do not give blind trust to anyone, period. I don't know about you but I wouldn't trust myself 100% of times and all the time. How many times have I promised myself to eat healthy and move more or change something only to repeatedly break my own promise. If I can't blindly trust myself 100% of the time how on earth do I hold someone else accountable to give me 100% trust worthiness AND GET IT 100% RIGHT?

If trust is based on getting it right, then you can't even trust yourself. An honest self-examination reveals that little separates us from others—that there's a bit of good in the worst of us and a bit of bad in the best of us. This is not the same as to stay with someone who is not willing to do whatever is necessary to be safe. However, we do want to live and experience life, and the price we pay for mistrust is disconnection from both self and others.

How do you know when it's safe to re-establish trust?
The importance of putting in the necessary effort to mend your trauma wounds following the betrayal and your partner's commitment to safety cannot be understated, ignored, or comprehended overnight. Even though you want to, it will be tough for you to trust them immediately after the hurt of the betrayal. However, if betrayal trauma is appropriately recognised and addressed by both partners, safe and trustworthy attachments can be formed.

But you may ask why would I want to trust the person who betrayed me so badly? This question has more than one answer. For some it is a matter of love and devotion. Some people do it to protect their finances or families. But every betrayed partner must have their own personal motivations for re-engaging or desiring to restore the relationship.

Your partner's repeated offences will only diminish your safety, increase your distrust and make re-building the relationship more challenging.

If your partner is just not getting it, take action before going any further with them. In these instances, your situation will be far too intricate and interconnected to improve over time. Unfortunately, the issues with a lack of actual recovery will only get worse with time, giving you and your loved ones more possibilities to experience future relapses and endure more suffering. Most of the time, unless sex addicts hit rock bottom, they won't simply take recovery seriously. Someone's rock bottom may be losing you or their family.

Obstacles to relational safety and trust:

- Sex addict isn't fully committed to the relationship or recovery.
- Inability of your SA partner to be truthful and honest. YOU BETTER RUN!
- The sex addict is not fully committed and engages in inconsistent sea saw recovery.
- The sex addict denies their lack of commitment and want you to get over it. There may still be some hope but enforce clear boundaries and do not give them endless chances.
- They are the 'I'm going to do it!' types who don't follow through on their pledges or words. Once again you need to employ clear boundaries without enabling them endless chances

Moving forward try and build what I call mindful trust which is formed once the betrayed partner consistently experiences alignment of the sex addict partner's words and actions. If you don't have a sense of safety, trust is ill-advised. By safety here, I mean that you believe you can continue to deal with the infidelity and your spouse without needing to control him or her and not feeling as if a surprise waits around every corner, because your mate is taking responsibility for their actions and is making efforts to stop the hurtful behaviour. To trust without safety is blind trust, which serves no good purpose except to enable someone you love to continue in hurtful behaviour and to open up yourself to a world of hurt.

You and your partner must continually focus on relationship restoration if you want to re-establish trust. Even though it may seem unjust, the betrayed partner must do a lot of the work to address their grief and trauma. Afterall, you have decided to go through the difficult grieving process in order to start over with the same partner that has betrayed you.

CHAPTER 8

What are triggers and when will they stop?

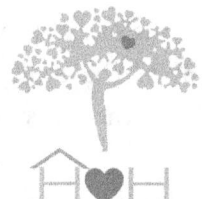

Strong emotional reactions are called triggers (or being triggered). These reactions go much beyond a simple uneasy sensation. When triggered, the betrayed partners experience a recurrence of their traumatic events. Betrayal trauma triggers occur when a similar circumstance, emotion, recollection, a person's actions, interactions, a movie, or a dream cause you to be reminded of the betrayal. When a person is triggered, their body goes into a flight, fight, freeze, or fawn response. Additionally, if the trauma isn't properly addressed, the betrayed partners will be forced to deal with their feelings in a destructive way.

A trigger may cause someone to feel nauseous, experience rapid and shallow breathing, or experience a rapid heart rate. On occasion, it can induce panic and a want to scream and run away. A trigger is the best input to activate the brain's alarm system. Triggers are a brain's protective mechanism established to prevent the betrayed partner from further harm. Unfortunately, betrayal trauma frequently puts the sufferers into overdrive, making it possible for them to be triggered frequently throughout the day. They may experience a constant sense of sorrow, grief, dread, fury, and/or rage as a result of this.

Even after the addict has attained sobriety and is following their recovery, the betrayed partner frequently still encounters a number of triggers. A trigger is a present-day reminder of the addict's destructive and addictive past behaviour. A trigger can be an intense emotional outburst that seems out of proportion to the situation, flashbacks to the addict's past behaviour, severe worry or panic, or a certain level of contempt for the addict.

The betrayed partner experiences several triggers shortly after the discovery or disclosure of sex addiction. Triggers are distressing and might appear out of nowhere. Occasionally, the betrayed partner does not become aware of being triggered until after the occurrence. Effective trauma therapy will provide both the betrayed partner and the sex addict the tools they need to manage the triggers. The betrayed partner first relies on the support of the sex addict partner in recovery (if the couple has decided to continue together) to aid them with trigger management until their acute trauma has subsided and they are ready to cope with their triggers on their own.

Triggers cause the trauma brain to split into two halves, one of which reacts to the present while the other reacts to the past experiences simultaneously. Triggers although very distressing and dysregulating for the betrayed partner, represent a normal feature of the recovery process from betrayal trauma and broken trust that has to be addressed, repaired and never ignored.

Trigger types - Any action taken by the recovering addict may act as a trigger, but environmental factors may also play a role. Triggers can include observing how an addict interacts with the other sex, finding them hiding anything on their phone or computer, or noticing they get home later than usual. Environmental triggers include seeing an explicit scene on television, seeing a massage parlour's flashing open sign, passing an adult bookstore, or hearing about an affair in a passing discussion.

These triggers can occasionally result in distrust and mistrust of the betrayed partner when patterns of action that were used to hide addiction are detected. For instance, if the addict had previously behaved out sexually while on work travels, travelling will likely operate as a trigger moving forwards. Indulging in late-night porn or other compulsive sexual behaviours can be a trigger for sex addicts, as can staying up late by themselves.

Other times, triggers are linked to the interplay of the intimate relationship that existed at the time of the addiction. If the sex addict's dysfunctional behaviours recurred, it's likely that a trigger response would be activated. For instance, if emotional detachment, or gaslighting were present around the actions of the addiction or if defensiveness or blame-shifting were used to cover up the addiction, these would induce a trigger response if repeated during recovery.

Relational patterns such as stonewalling, avoidant behaviours after a disagreement, and anger outbursts or extreme fury may have been employed in the past as a means of hiding or diverting attention from the addictive behaviour. If they keep happening, they can activate the trauma brain and serve as a reminder of the betrayed partner's experience, cause emotional dysregulation and induce triggers.

As was previously indicated, triggers frequently result in intense emotional responses, including fits of fury or avoidance. They could send the betrayed spouse into a downward cycle of pessimism and despair, which might lead to a relapse of safety-seeking behaviours. These include pacifying oneself with food, extended screen time, compulsive shopping, excessive drinking, or other compulsive habits, or by acting as a detective sifting through emails and text messages.

Some triggers, like the aforementioned travel trigger, are simpler to plan for. Triggers, though, frequently strike suddenly. You can be better prepared for unplanned and unforeseen triggers if you have a plan in place for how you and your partner will react to them. The best results are obtained when the couple manages triggers together. In these situations, the recovered addict must acknowledge, validate, reassure and show empathy rather than defending themselves or making the trigger about them. By spending time with the betrayed partner, allowing them to process their emotions, responding to them when they are ready to re-engage, and offering **co-regulation** (*Co-regulation involves a range of healthy responses, such as a warm, soothing manner, a gentle tone of voice, verbal validation, and providing emotional and physical safety*) through sincere affirmation, they can assist in deactivating the trauma brain.

It would be ineffective for the sex addict to be moping around, unhappy, impatient, resentful, pushing the betrayed partner to move on getting over the triggers, or informing the betrayed partner that triggers are inappropriate because they have recovered and are no longer sex addicts.

When would triggers stop?

Every hurt partner experiences this differently, and there is no set timeframe. Triggers are the unwanted gifts of betrayal caused by sex addiction, and they will continue to give for a very long time. According to my clinical observations, triggers will disappear more quickly if recovering addicts show compassion, validation and provide co-regulation to the betrayed partner. Triggers can vanish more quickly if the sufferer feels confident expressing and sharing their emotions in the relationship. It is also possible, though, that years or even decades after the betrayal, the traumatized partner may still occasionally find themselves the target of a trigger. There is no one solution that fits all. However, rest assure that as the healing process advances, triggers will lessen in frequency and duration.

One betrayed partner's account of her triggers is as follows:

> *They frequently arrive as expected or unexpected, but they always do. If I let them stay or stay longer, they always stay longer. Sometimes I'm awful about my triggers because if I let my guards down they managed to bring me down fast. Although it's entirely up to me and my choices, I've learnt to replace those negative or displeased thoughts that triggers bring with gratitude and appreciations. I'm far more likely to be triggered- remember the pain- until I've made progress on my healing journey or feel safe once more. At the same time I am all too aware of how challenging and bothersome these triggers are. For the time being, I simply let my intrusive ideas come but do not try to entertain them. I can now sit with triggers and keep telling myself that I'm safe because I recognise that they are a part of my journey. To get to this point, I had to go through a bloody long process and spend many hours in therapy. It is not easy.*

Sarah, divorced wife of a sex addict

CHAPTER 9

Why polygraph?

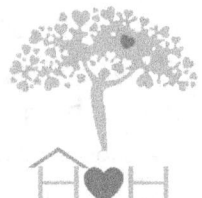

The discovery of a lie will always hurt more and deeper than the disclosure of the bitter truth.

Although sex addicts lie and manipulate sincerely, they may not always do so with malice or malicious intent. Their constant need for chemicals to soothe the survival centre of their brain, which addiction has hijacked, is what drives their lies.

In sex addicts' brain the prefrontal cortex's logical, compassionate, and empathetic functions are suppressed as the primitive limbic system seeks out chemicals (in this case, sex or compulsive sexual behaviours) at any expense. The demand for mood-altering or mind-altering chemicals are driven by the addict's most fundamental need, which is to survive. And lying to everyone who gets in the way of them getting their fix they so desperately want is part of it. No one is more likely to be manipulated by an addict than the partners.

After being discovered, one method an addict manipulates is by making little confessions of wrongdoing to a partner to hide larger lies and other betrayal.

Additionally, addicts may deceive by placing the shame and blame for their actions on another person or by making empty promises to seek help. The manner that the lies characterise the betrayal as premeditated, calculated, hidden, spiteful, thoughtless, and personal is one aspect that contributes to the agony of betrayal trauma that causes such deep wounds. Even after being told that sex addiction is not about them, the betrayed partner may find it difficult to accept this explanation since the pain of being deceived is seen to be so deeply personal. How can a partner tell if an addict is being truthful in the disclosure or still trying to hide something, especially after years and years of lying? Following what could seem like another confessional when the partner's trust reserves are exhausted and their instincts are deemed to be unreliable, a polygraph examination might be a helpful tool. In my practise, I regularly run into several sex addicts who confess that if it weren't for the polygraph exam, they would carry some of their secrets with them to the grave.

In my most recent study, only female partners of sex addict men who asked their partners to take a polygraph test acknowledged knowing the complete truth, while other women who did not request such a test were still unaware of the whole depth of their partners' compulsive behaviours. A polygraph test is valuable when one's sense of security and self is severely shaken by sexual betrayal and lying, and this can lead one to doubt their own sense of reality. Additionally, studies have indicated that compared to other types

Why polygraph?

of trauma, betrayal trauma is linked to higher somatic symptoms and mistrust because betrayal wounds penetrate the human psyche deeply. Therefore, building safety and trust is crucial if the relationship is to survive and if the partner is to recover.

In the early phases of recovery, more and more couples are discovering that rigors interventions like polygraph testing can help them build a foundation of safety, trust and accountability if the test is carefully and therapeutically prepared for. The tests must be administered by a certified polygraph examiner who is familiar with delivering and analysing polygraph data and who upholds by the stringent ethical standards established by recognised polygraph associations like the American Polygraph Association (APA). Founded in 1966, the APA is the foremost organisation in the world devoted to the use of scientific approaches supported by evidence for evaluating credibility.

A polygraph measures physiological changes, including variations in electrodermal skin resistance, blood pressure, blood volume, and breathing (both inhalation and exhalation). It is essentially analysing physiological changes in the body at the start of a pertinent question regarding a particular activity, albeit it is a little more sophisticated than that.

I frequently encounter sex addicts who are reluctant to be completely honest and who impose manipulations by either disputing the validity of the test after failing it or simply refusing to take it. Unfortunately, some partners still have naiveté and are in denial about their partner's honesty, so they continue to believe them. Such betrayed partners will never know if the sex addict is still engaging in compulsive behaviours. As a result, those sex addicts who don't take a polygraph test learn how to mislead and conceal their acting out behaviours more effectively to avoid being detected.

A polygraph examination consists of the pre-test interview, the polygraph test, and the analysis of the results. Pre-test interview is essentially a conversation between the sex addict and the polygrapher. This document's goal is to inform and familiarise the addict with the procedures, goals, resources, and questions related to the test.

The examination itself, which takes up the second section, asks pertinent questions about the addict's involvement in the compulsive sexual behaviour under consideration. All questions are straightforward, devoid of legal language or confusing language and uncomplicated and issues are kept separated from each other. Every question is dealt with a distinct behavioural problem.

The third stage of the polygraph compares the addict's responses to the pertinent questions to their control questions. A few polygraph tests are available. One is known as the disclosure polygraph, and it is normally administered immediately following the completion of all disclosures. After that, a few months later, and then once a year to assess ongoing sobriety. Some persons might need additional testing, depending on the level of deception or relapse rates.

When it comes to believing the truth from a sex addict, I typically tell betrayed partners that I still believe the polygraph test. After all, sex addicts are expert liars, and the polygraph test was developed with a single, clear purpose in mind: to uncover deception. An effective way to put a stop to years of secrets is with a polygraph, which can help the relationship begin to mend.

A polygraph test is a great choice for re-establishing psychological and emotional safety and removes at least some of the ambiguity. Honesty and empathy are the two most important tools the betrayed partners need at the beginning of their healing. Being

Why polygraph?

honest and letting a polygraph verify the sex addict's honesty is the proper course of action. When used appropriately, a polygraph is a trustworthy tool that can offer some hope to both the addict and the betrayed partner. The addict should also think of the test as a gift they voluntarily provide to their betrayed partner in order to establish a solid foundation of trust. Furthermore, over the years, those who have taken polygraph tests have confided in me that, once they get over their initial nervousness, the test becomes one of their best motivators and helps them advance in their sobriety. They may find it to be of tremendous assistance in maintaining their sobriety and mending their relationships. Since it causes the addicts to feel nervous, the first polygraph can typically be challenging. In my own clinical practise, when given the option, the majority of couples decide to incorporate polygraph testing into a safety or therapy plan. Most couples understand their advantages for themselves and their relationship.

It just takes one untruth to cast doubt on all truths.

Advantages of polygraph testing for betrayed partners:

- Outlines a useful method for discovering the truth.
- Gives early recovery work a greater sense of accountability.
- Confirms what is already known and identifies the unknowns to assist in restoring one's sense of intuition.
- It protects against inaccuracies and further harmful lies when done in conjunction with a therapeutic disclosure.
- Once they are aware of the reality, the betrayed partner can begin the healing process.
- Confirms the partner's intuition and gives the betrayed partner confidence that they weren't crazy.

- Creates a sense of physical, mental and sexual safety.
- Demonstrates the amount to which the addict is willing to be open and truthful about their compulsive behaviours, their dedication to recovery or even lack of such commitment.
- It lowers made-up stories by getting rid of the behaviours that the partner might have thought were involved.
- It restores some control to the betrayed partner, allowing them to choose how much of the truth they want to know.
- If the betrayed partner decides to stay in the relationship, it offers safety because they know what to look for.
- Prevents repeated disclosures, which would re-traumatize the betrayed partner.
- Without the test the betrayed partner is left to trust an addict who initially doesn't have the skills to disclose the whole truth.

Advantages of polygraph testing for the sex addict:

- Gives them a way to start rebuilding their relationship's trust with their partner.
- Rebuilding the relational trust by trusting the betrayed partner with the whole truth.
- It is a useful technique to rule out actions that the person may be accused of engaging in.
- Presents a disclosure that has been carefully examined and written.
- If done correctly, it can serve as a process of de-shaming where the addict purges all of their secrets and lies and begins their journey towards liberation from addiction.

Why polygraph?

- A therapeutic test serve a couple the ground zero where the addict can practise being real in their relationship.
- Helps one become more accountable to themselves, their partners, and sobriety process.
- Provides support and credibility to the sex addict in the event that the betrayed partner is triggered and starts to question if the whole truth been reported.
- It prevents the sex addict from controlling, manipulating or gaslighting the betrayed partner or the process anymore.
- Accelerates the healing process by being upfront about the extent of acting out behaviours from the beginning.
- The only tool accessible to an addict to force them to consistently practise being honest.

Reliability and accuracy of polygraph test

Keep in mind that people perform polygraphs, and just like with surgeons, therapists, and educators, there are competent polygraphers and less competent ones. However, if your polygrapher is competent and has some expertise dealing with sex addiction/ betrayal trauma, you should get results that are 98–99 % accurate or higher. Many times, sex addicts themselves or other less qualified therapists in the field of sex addiction oppose such tests and question their reliability for a variety of reasons. These include the fact that the addict does not want to be forced to reveal a lifetime of deceit and compulsive sexual behaviours. Additionally, sex addiction and betrayal trauma are relatively new fields, and many therapists who claim to be knowledgeable about working with these two groups actually have no idea how to support either the addict or their partners. When couples complain that they wasted time and money on non-specialist therapist who did more harm than good, professionals like me are frequently left to pick up the pieces.

To betrayed partners and well-intentioned therapists, I ask the following question: Who or what can be trusted more? Who is more likely to be lying: a sex addict or this scientific test that was specifically created and engineered to detect deception? Alcoholics can use a breathalyser, however we are all aware that these tools are not always 100% accurate, but we don't argue with them. We chose not to cast doubt on urine and other drug testing techniques for drug addicts, despite the fact that they are not 100% accurate. But everyone appears to be insisting that a polygraph test must be 100% accurate in order to be acceptable for use in detecting deception (anything close to 100% is not good enough and renders the test unreliable?). This is illogical and a further insult to the integrity of betrayed partners who have gone through a great deal of pain and deserve some clarity.

I always go with the test since, up to now, it hasn't let down my betrayed partners or sex addicts and has significantly helped undo the harm that repeated lies have created. It has also been the only international measure for monitoring the continued honesty and sobriety of sex addicts. It has been used for decades in other countries, such as the USA.

A polygraph test preparation also involves a lot of ongoing assessment on my part as a competent sex addict specialist. More often than not, I can tell who is still lying and who has disclosed honestly, so the test frequently verifies what I have previously determined. So far there haven't been any failures in my clinical work where it hasn't turned out that the addicts either lied or withheld information, and there haven't been any instances of sincere addicts failing the test either.

Since a sex addict is a good liar (due to years of practice), betrayed partners have long told me they are reluctant to believe a polygraph. What if the addict can fool the test? This may be true, and it is undoubtedly distressing. The harsh reality is that while the addicts have perfected the art of fooling their partners and others through years of deception and dishonesty, it will be very challenging for them to execute the same skill in a polygraph test and with a knowledgeable polygrapher.

A polygraph is but one element in the recovery and healing processes. Even if the addict takes the polygraph and does well on it, there will still be severe problems if they are still acting callously and showing no remorse or empathy for what they have done to their partner.

The polygraph test is extremely sensitive to lying or keeping secrets. For example, if a sex addict is aware of past activities that could affect their partner or relationship but choose not to share them. Even though the polygraph test's questions have nothing to do with those situations, they fail because the addict continues to tell lies and conceal important information from their betrayed partner.

Courts do not allow the use of polygraphs.
Based on following facts, this is definitely the biggest myth regarding polygraphs being admissible in court. In certain countries, candidates for important positions in the public or private sectors as well as criminal suspects are questioned using polygraphs. The **FBI** (Federal Bureau of Investigation), **DEA** (Drug Enforcement Administration), **CIA** (Central Intelligence Agency), **NSA** (National Security Agency), as well as different police departments like the **LAPD** (Los Angeles Police Department) and the Virginia State Police use

polygraph tests to question suspects or screen potential employees. Within the US federal government, a polygraph test is often referred to as a psychophysiological detection of deception **(PDD)** test.

Polygraphs can be used at different stages of a trial, despite the fact that state rules in the USA vary. A Grand Jury commonly uses them to determine whether to send a person to trial. Although there is some disagreement between the defence and prosecution lawyers on the quantity and nature of evidence that will be allowed in court, a polygraph serves as a sort of evidence. In some cases, judge's order polygraph tests so that the results can be presented as evidence in court. Additionally, although not always employed in criminal situations, polygraph examinations are frequently used in cases of theft or fraud. They can also be used to resolve legal matters such as dispute, insurance issues, and personal injury claims.

A polygraph test is reportedly often conducted on paramedics, police officers, firefighters, and state troopers in the United States, according to a 2018 article in Wired magazine.

When a polygraph test is used in England and Wales, the results cannot be used as evidence in court. To monitor serious sexual offenders on parole in England and Wales, however, the Offender Management Act of 2007 established a polygraph monitoring option; these tests were made mandatory for high risk sexual offenders on parole in England and Wales in 2014 (Bowcott, 2014).

Currently, Belgium is the nation in Europe where police utilise polygraph testing the most frequently, conducting roughly 300 tests yearly as part of criminal investigations. Although the outcomes have been used in jury trials, they are not being used as evidence in bench trials (Meijer, 2017).

Why polygraph?

In Lithuania, where polygraphs have been used since 1992, law enforcement utilises the Event Knowledge Test, a modification of the Concealed Information Test, during criminal investigations (Saldžiunas & Kovalenko, 2008).

Some therapists and clients assert that polygraph results could result in a false positive, meaning the individual could tell the truth but the polygraph would detect a lie. I have never seen this happen in my experience. Although it is incredibly rare, I am not suggesting it never happens. Additionally, people will claim that a person can pass the polygraph if they think a lie is true; this is also quite uncommon.

I would never advocate using polygraph testing to replace developing an intuition or a capacity to detect dishonest behaviour. However, polygraph testing might aid in providing greater clarity up until the point where one has recovered from the years of disorientation brought on by persistent manipulation, gaslighting, and deception.

Please be aware that a polygraph is not in any way administered as a punishment, but rather as a powerful and useful tool for re-establishing relational safety and trust.

According to research on the use of polygraphs in the treatment of sex addiction, 46.7% of partners found the results to be a confirmation of what their partner had already disclosed, 20.7% said the results had helped them regain their trust in their partner, and 26.7% said the results had improved their relationship (Manning, 2022).

Although polygraph testing is an option, I highly urge couples to consider it as they develop their safety and healing plans. To ask a recovered addict to undergo a polygraph test is a relatively small act of atonement after the ongoing history of lying and associated harm is clearly acknowledged.

CHAPTER 10

Grief and loss induced by betrayal trauma

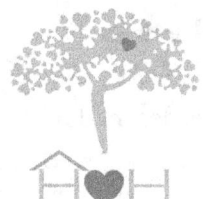

Betrayal trauma can be very difficult to understand and can be very complex. There could be a variety of emotions involved, including hurt, confusion, betrayal, and outrage. People who have experienced trauma brought on by betrayal frequently go through a number of stages of grieving and loss, even if every person's experience is unique. Various grief associated feelings may come to betrayed partners at any point during the grieving process and not necessarily in the sequence they might expect. Everyone has a different grief process, therefore it's possible that not every betrayed partner will necessarily go through all the different feelings and experiences associated with different phases. How a person grieves can be influenced by a variety of factors, including the severity and circumstances of the loss, individual differences in attitude and character, and cultural, spiritual, and religious beliefs.

Grief is incredibly individualised. It's not really organised or logical. It doesn't adhere to any timetables or plans. You can feel sad, angry, isolated, or emptied. All of these occurrences are normal and correct. Although everyone grieves in their own way, there are certain similarities among the phases and sequence of emotions that are felt throughout mourning. According to Kübler-Ross's grief model, the five stages of grief are: shock and denial, anger, bargaining, depression and acceptance. The betrayal trauma's loss and grief phases are:

1. Shock and denial phase

At this point, you first have learned of the betrayal and find it hard to accept that it actually has occurred. The sensation that you are dreaming or that everything will be fine when you wake up may be your primary experienced. You are at the shock stage as soon as you become aware of your partner's betrayal and deception. You go into a condition of fight, flight, freeze, or fawn, feeling numb and wondering how you're going to make it through the day. Grief brought on by the trauma of betrayal can be a potent feeling. It's normal to reject the loss caused by the shock and act as though it isn't real in order to cope with the strong and frequently unexpected emotions generated by the acute transgressions of sex addiction. If you reject the occurrence, you will have more time to gradually take in the information and begin to comprehend it. This is a typical defensive tactic that decreases the effect of the stressful experience. Depending on how severe the betrayal has been, this stage may remain a few days or even weeks. Additionally, you can

Grief and loss induced by betrayal trauma

experience a sense of apathy (lack of excitement, desire, or concern) and disconnection from the world. It can be very daunting and perplexing during this phase.

Some betrayed partners become quiet and withdrawn, shut off, and isolated and are unable to carry out routine daily tasks. Others can't control their emotions, may become aggressive, display explosive anger, and might attack their partners and others when emotionally distressed. To assist the person in dealing with the intense suffering and discomfort, the shock and denial phase acts as an anaesthetic and numbing agent.

The shock is so overpowering that what keeps you alive and allows you to survive the betrayal is denying the loss. You can feel at this moment that life and everything else you once treasured are useless and meaningless at this time.

It can be quite challenging for relatives and friends trying to support you through the denial period if they are unfamiliar with grieving and its phases. They might even make an effort to defend or rationalize the betrayal, or they might simply completely disregard it. The detective work done by the betrayed partner as a safety seeking strategy and an effort to uncover the truth is the significant element of this phase.

This stage of grief is extremely startling because it may involve re-traumatizing incidents because there may be further discoveries and the sex addict often continues to lie and gradually drip-feeds the betrayed partner with half-truths. As a result, the betrayed partner feels compelled to spend a lot of time dwelling over the specifics of the betrayal in an effort to piece together a coherent narrative of it. Most sufferers isolate themselves in the interim, which exacerbates their emotional pain and distress. I compare this stage for the betrayed partner to a zombie-like and out-of-body state. When the betrayed partner must continue to carry out necessary professional or daily obligations while going through the dreadful shock and denial phase of their loss, it is an added insult and further trauma.

2. Anger phase

Despite being a normal and healthy feeling to feel, anger is misunderstood by many people. Naturally, you'll become upset when you sense danger. Being betrayed partners typically express their fury by explosion, suppression, or a combination of both during the anger phase of grief since the central nervous system is so overtaxed therefor, trauma brain is constantly stimulated and activated. This phase is marked by the body's fight-or-flight reaction, a survival instinct. The adrenaline rush causes your heart rate to accelerate, your blood pressure to rise, and you to become more vigilant. Anger frequently drives intense, even aggressive feelings that are all defence-related actions because you feel threatened by the betrayal and the person that betrayed you. This is the phase where you begin to verbally communicate the hurt and rage you are feeling. Although anger is a normal reaction to feeling unsafe, as already mentioned, if this stage is left unattended, it can be deeply disturbing and linger for weeks or even months. It is typical for anger to be directed inward (against oneself) or outward—to your sex addict partner, friends, relatives, kids, or even total strangers.

Anger must be felt for a while as the body heals. Anger is a secondary emotion that appears to cover up more fragile emotions underlying it. Pain and fear are often the underlying causes of anger. It's crucial to allow yourself to feel the anger while keeping in mind that pain and, even deeper, fear lie beneath anger. Redefining anger as fear underneath the pain might help you get to the bottom of the issue

Grief and loss induced by betrayal trauma

fast rather than becoming bogged down in draining resentments. Ask yourself and pause: *What is the pain that has surfaced, and what am I fearful of? What boundaries have been violated for me to feel the pain and be fearful here and now?*

Self-regulation is really beneficial and slows down the trauma brain so that you may express your anger more effectively. Nevertheless, if you are in the early stages of your grieving, it may be naturally very difficult to do so.

Initially you will be a mess and that's ok.

Your healing process will be hampered, and you'll become more bitter if you try to suppress your anger. If you reclaim your powers by allowing yourself to feel the anger, you will start to heal more quickly and effectively.

If you can feel your pain, then you can heal your pain.

As a betrayed partner, going through the anger phase gives you the strength and tenacity you need to deal with the practical challenges that come up while you're grieving. This could include the determination to uphold new clear boundaries and consequences, make challenging decisions, or supply the necessary energy if a separation is required.

While there is a short-term survival advantage to being angry, it's crucial to realise that this advantage quickly disappears. Don't deceive yourself by continuing to hold on to it since your brain is now dependent on the adrenaline rush you get whenever you are angry. If you don't deliberately recognise and break this destructive cycle, it can be tough for you to escape this new addiction. Additionally, constantly keep in mind that you must be the recipient of this respect, therefore learn to express your anger in a respectable way. It is possible for the betrayed partner to become so out of control during the anger phase that things get violent, people get hurt, children suffer trauma, neighbours get involved, and the police may even be called. No matter how severely one has been traumatised or grieving, this is incredibly harmful and can be avoided. This is not fair on anyone, but most especially it is not fair on you who have experienced so much suffering. Many betrayed partners have confided in me that they feel disappointed and ashamed of how they expressed their anger. If you can't keep yourself or others safe, please take some time off and temporarily disengage while working with a therapist until you can vent your anger in a less damaging way. If you are able to express and manage your anger in a constructive manner, you will be able to assert the self-respect you wish to maintain.

3. Bargaining phase

At this phase, you can find yourself attempting to lessen or rectify your loss by bargaining with your surroundings, destiny, God/higher power, yourself, and others. According to the American Psychological Association, the bargaining stage of grief is a time when you may attempt to make a deal with yourself or a God/higher power in an effort to reverse the loss (APA, 2013).

Bargaining is another strategy for coping with the feelings of grief and assists you to temporary put off the depression, uncertainty, or pain. In this phase, one engages in mental haggling to justify choices that might have been made differently or more successfully to prevent the loss. Bargaining can take the form of statements like:

Grief and loss induced by betrayal trauma

- *If only I had been thinner or sexier, he wouldn't have needed to go elsewhere to be sexually satisfied.*
- *If I had trusted my instincts and didn't believe him last year when he was lying, I wouldn't feel like a fool today.*
- *If I had more sex with him instead of being so busy with the kids, he wouldn't have betrayed me.*
- *If I had been more persistent every time he came home late and checked his phone more frequently, I might have been able to stop the betrayal.*
- *Maybe I shouldn't have encouraged him when he wanted to include porn into our relationship.*

The betrayed partner uses bargaining as a means of coping with the sense of helplessness that follows a loss brought on by betrayal. It occurs when you find it difficult to accept both the consequences of your sex addict partner's actions and the limits of your own attempts to control the situation. The bargaining stage gives a way to restore control when the betrayed partner feels as though everything is spiralling out of control. Even though these agreements or contracts can't be upheld, by highlighting what you could have done better, they provide a sense of increased control.

Those who practise religion or other forms of spirituality may genuinely bargain with God. The betrayed partner attempts to haggle with God, or the universe in the bargaining phase. This stage, which can endure for weeks or months, usually include vowing never to commit any specific offences again or asking for the sex addict to make things right. *If you make this reality go away, I will pray more and be more devoted to my faith*, or *If you don't punish him for the betrayal, I will quit worshipping you*, are examples of religious bargaining. For those around the betrayed partners, this stage can be quite frustrating because the healing process is often delayed as a result.

The grief process bargaining stage is characterised by the features listed below:

- Regrets or feelings of shame about your language or behaviour.
- Fantasizing, wishing or praying for a different reality.
- Persistent anxiety, uncertainty, or fearfulness.
- Speculating on and obsessing on potential different outcomes.
- Taking personal responsibility and feeling guilty.
- Self-condemnation.
- Stressing and over analysing things to the point of exhaustion.
- Increased self-criticism and judgement of others, especially the sex addict partner.
- Comparing your situation to others.
- Becoming future focused and imagining the worst.
- Lack of self-compassion and forgiving.

You must understand that the bargaining phase is a normal aspect of your grief process in order to manage it effectively. Through bargaining, you may keep your hope alive—something you'll need to do to get through your loss and pain. As you begin to accept reality as it is, you will gradually stop engaging in this inclination. Try to obtain some perspective and emotionally distance yourself from the negative thoughts rather than letting them consume your thinking. It may be helpful to discuss these concerns with a trustworthy and safe individual who can aid in your processing. It is what it is, repeat it to yourself aloud. You start making changes in your life that are more supportive of your progress when you decide to shift your perspective from trying to change reality or everything that is beyond your control to accepting the bitter reality and everything that you can control. At this point, you will be most capable of moving past the bargaining phases. Journaling your feelings, goals, and commitments and meditating on them may help you become more self-aware and conscious of your true feelings and reasons behind them rather than getting lost in them.

It's crucial to get support from a mental health professional who is experienced with grieving related to sex addiction. Although this grieving process is similar to general grieving and loss, it is quite different, and not everyone can comprehend it or support you through it. You could also take comfort in betrayed partner-based grief support groups (Dr. Douglas Weiss, for example, runs a number of Facebook support groups for betrayed partners). Please be careful that some Facebook groups portray the hurt partner as a co-dependent or co-addict. These derogatory views and perspectives are subtly imposed, and they have the potential to severely re-traumatize and re-victimize the betrayed partners.

With time, your suffering should become more bearable, and you could find it easier to accept events beyond your control. However, grieving can be incredibly difficult for some betrayed partners for a long time following a loss. Be patient with yourself.

4. Sadness and depression phase

After the phase of bargaining, your attention returns to the here and now. For you, the betrayed partner you may feel like giving up on the things you formerly cared about since everything looks dismal and gloomy. You could find it difficult to get out of bed and go about your day the way you used to because you feel unmotivated and overburdened. When empty sensations start to surface, you realise how deeply grief has impacted your life. This depressive phase appears to go on forever. Realizing that this depression is not a sign of a mental condition is crucial. However, this phase can exacerbate pre-existing symptoms of depression or induce long-lasting depressive episodes. Many betrayed partners may need to consult with their doctors and find out if they need to take medication during this phase.

It is the appropriate response to your significant loss. You can withdraw from life and lose yourself in intense grief. If recovering from grief is a process, one of the many necessary benchmarks along the way is processing the sadness and depression. Again, you're not alone; these emotions are all common and essential to the grieving process.

Contrary to popular belief, people don't go through the phases of grieving in sequence or even one at a time. The betrayed partner may go through all phases of the grieving process, or they may not go through all of them but some. The frequency of occurrence, the severity, the duration, and the symptoms that go along with each phase can all differ.

This stage can appear to some betrayed partners like a persistent, oppressive fog. They may perceive life as depressing, burdensome, and isolating. Their entire focus is on developing the motivation to go on. This phase can be extremely crippling and frequently results in suicidal ideas or self-harm behaviours.

In the phase of sadness and depression, the betrayed partner could feel:

- Depressed, lifeless, drained, uninspired, hopelessness, low energy and worn out.
- A lack of joy.
- There is no way out of your grief.
- Weighed down by the demands of daily life.
- The need for excessive sleep or insomnia.
- Inability to stop crying.
- A wave of melancholy accompanies every memory.
- That others don't grasp their loss.
- Fearful that others won't cope with their grief.
- The desire for self-isolation instead of seeking the comfort of a community.

For the depressive phase of grief to be managed, it is essential to accept support from friends, relatives, co-workers, spiritual leaders, and other trustworthy and safe individuals. Depression symptoms are frequently made worse by withdrawing from people and isolating oneself. Allow yourself to experience all of your feelings. There are no bad feelings since they are all present to communicate with you about who you are and what you need to do. Put your attention on accepting all of your feelings. If you wait for your feelings to motivate you to do action while you're depressed or unhappy, you might as well wait forever. Instead, you must push yourself to take action and the feelings of motivations will follow. Healthy routines and practices such as walking, therapy, journaling, praying, yoga, meditation or simply playing with a pet are beneficial for triggering feelings of accomplishment, or purpose. Additionally, asking for or needing support is acceptable, common, and even important. Reach out, do it now and not later.

5. Acceptance phase

Although acceptance can alter the perspective through which you view the previous phases, it frequently comes and goes, and you can even experience it while still attempting to get past other stages like anger and sadness. You are in the acceptance phase as the betrayed partner if you have finally accepted what has happened. Even if you don't like or agree with your reality, you can now accept that the betrayal happened and there is nothing you can do to change it, making it easier for you to go about your daily activities than it was in the earlier stages.

This phase may be very liberating and typically leads to a deeper understanding of who you are while acknowledging your new reality. Despite the fact that it may be challenging, this phase is eventually healing because you are less involved in constructing fantasies about how you want things to have turned out.

Accepting that the past is gone and that you need to reset your perspective by living in the here and now . You cease attempting to recover what was lost once you realise that you can never replace what was lost but you can consciously create another life. Acceptance involves realising and embracing that the healing process will be challenging or even messy at times. Nevertheless, you continue on, regaining control over your life and moving forward with authority.

Acceptance does not mean that you are not able to experience suffering, loss, or misfortune. It suggests that you are aware that stress-free, easy living was never a promise. It requires acknowledging what you are going through, validating yourself while doing so, having self-compassion, and recalibrating yourself with the present state. It involves staying mindful and maintaining an open, inquisitive mindset to prevent getting stuck in the grieving process, which can be beneficial for your healing journey.

Acceptance fosters self-love and self-compassion and may look as follows:

- You are becoming more knowledgeable about sex addiction, betrayal trauma, and seeing probable explanations for your partner's actions.
- Realizing that you no longer have relational trust and accepting that fact may be considered acceptance.
- Acceptance could entail ending the relationship or separating. Because not all relationships can be saved, especially when only one person is willing to put in the effort and make the necessary changes.
- Acceptance may mean accepting your own obligations and boundaries while continuing to hold your partner accountable for the betrayal.
- The goal of acceptance is to integrate the past into the present without letting it control how you will evolve in the future.
- Recognising when you are self-critical and aiming your resentment and displeasure about what is happening on yourself. You then identify, express your anger, clarify what it really means, and take action to alleviate it.
- Checking in with yourself and taking some time to reflect on your requirements and current state. Accepting that self-care of is a necessity, not a luxury, and that neglecting your needs in favour of others or your work it will hamper your healing and lead to burnout.
- Instead of dragging the past with you, you are more present-focused and mindful.

The betrayed partner may experience frequent ups and downs in their emotions, ideas, attitudes, and behaviours even throughout the accepting phase. It can be difficult to maintain acceptance when a sex addict regularly exhibits inappropriate sexual behaviour, relapses, displays other flaws, or lacks empathy and validation for the betrayed partner.

Betrayed partners in my recent research described the following deep losses brought on by the obsessive sexual behaviours of sex addicts. How many resonate with you?

> **The betrayed partners in my research described a number of losses that deeply grieved them. Here are the reported losses of:**
>
> - Their self-identity as a lover and a partner.
> - The partners' character as they had understood it.
> - Their past reality.
> - The life they had come to know.
> - A lack of faith in a stable future together.
> - Their emotional stability due to the possibility of relapse by their male partner, or even their unwillingness to cease sex addiction.
> - Relational commitment. Most people consider fidelity sacred.
> - The sacredness of togetherness in a committed dyad that meant separation from others appeared to be lost for the affected women in this study.
> - Confidence in people and relationships (i.e., family members, friends and various other relationships, such as those with themselves, or their god/higher power).

Grief and loss induced by betrayal trauma

- Their past sexual openness, which is now hampered by intrusive thoughts, self-doubts, and the incapacity to compete with the images or people with whom their male partner interacted.
- Financial security.
- A more carefree interpersonal dynamic (with their partners and others).
- Their usual family system.
- Health due to the physical, sexual, and emotional ailments.
- Spiritual security or identity, even the loss of trust in a higher power.
- Of relational trust.
- The future they envisioned.
- Trust for self, others, and god/higher power.
- Your sense of self.

CHAPTER 11

Should you stay or should you go?

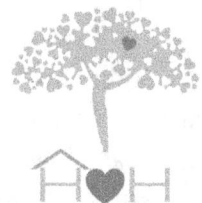

There is such a high level of emotion after learning what your sex addict partner has done, while you are also dealing with a lot of uncertainties. You must carefully weigh all the relevant factors before deciding whether to continue the relationship or call it quits. It makes sense that the shock you're feeling would cloud your judgement and make things unclear. It goes without saying that you should think about your children's wellbeing and feelings if you have any. Try to put yourself in a better stable and safe situation before addressing the difficult decision of whether to continue the relationship with your spouse or end it. While you're taking care of yourself and dealing with the initial shock, it's quite acceptable if you temporarily need some distance from your sex addict partner. It's critical that each person has realistic expectations and is aware of what it means to remain in a relationship with a sex addict before considering any justifications for continuing the relationship. The basic fact is that addiction frequently never completely goes away. The addict might reach a point when they are comfortable and feel more in control than ever, but in reality, they are still recovering addicts. Recovery is an ongoing process that differs from person to person and is not a quick fix. Even if your sex addict partner receives therapy, keep in mind that not everyone is equipped to deal with sex addiction in a relationship. You have every right to leave your partner if you so want. Never assume responsibility for what they do since you need to first look after your own mental health.

One challenging component of sexual addiction is the shame and secrecy associated with it. Sex addiction appears to be stigmatised in contrast to drug or alcohol addiction. Because it undermines the sacredness of intimate relationships, and therefore it appears to be the bad apple of addictions. The added stress caused by needing to be more covert might intensify feelings of guilt and shame. As a result, restraining urges become more difficult, and behaviours become unpredictable. Due to their warped perceptions of sex, sex addicts lose interest in intimacy with a real partner. Thus, women and people begin to be viewed as just objects to be lusted after. At this point, the betrayed partner must choose the unpleasant reality of the addiction and whether to remain with the sex addict and work through recovery with them or leave because they are unable to accept what has happened.

Here are a few succinct accounts to help you decide what to do when you're ready.

Should you stay or should you go?

Your reasons to stay:

- You are aware of what recovery entails and your own work you need to do.
- You're willing to take into account your partner's recovery needs.
- Both of you are still committed to restoring the relationship.
- Your partner wants to recover from their sex addiction and accepts responsibility for their behaviour.
- Your desire to be together and you are committed to healthy communication.
- You are both ready to be respectful of one another and make new experiences.
- You both have similar future objectives and are prepared to collaborate with one another to accomplish them.
- Undoubtedly, you would be losing a really valuable person or relationship if you weren't together.
- You are unsure of your motivation for leaving.
- Your sex addict partner is working consistently to respect the boundaries and repairs the past wounds.
- You both think that eventually, your relationship could get stronger.

Your reasons to leave:

- Your sex addict partner denies their addiction.
- Your partner refuses to take ownership of their sex addiction or start true recovery.
- The root of your partner's sex addiction is something they won't address.
- In your relationship violence or domestic abuse has occurred.
- You are unwilling to participate in healing and recovery processes.
- The discovery/disclosure came at a time when the relationship was ending any way.
- You're unable or unwilling to forgive and reconcile with your partner.
- Your partner is unable or unwilling to maintain a safe relationship.
- Your partner has engaged in unlawful behaviour, and you are unable or unwilling to support them.
- Your partner is unwilling to give up certain affair partner.
- Your sex addict partner is no longer someone you respect or like, or vice versa.
- You're staying just because you're scared of what people may say if you left.
- Because you're afraid of being by yourself, you're simply waiting till you've met someone else.

CHAPTER 12

What are boundaries and why are they essential for individual healing and relationship restoration?

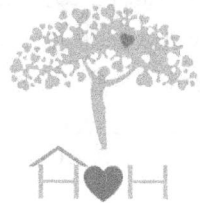

What are boundaries and why are they essential for individual healing and relationship restoration?

A line that denotes the limits of a zone; a dividing line, is how the Oxford Dictionary (2010) defines a boundary. According to the definition of boundary, what people do to you shows their values and who they are, just as how you allow people to treat you reveals your values and who you are.

Setting boundaries is done so that the betrayed partner may look after themselves. It's about coming to know yourself better, loving and respecting yourself more. If you never have to establish boundaries, you will never discover your true self, free yourself from the grip of co-dependency, and come to terms with what is healthy for you.

The betrayed partner is commonly the subject and target of all the sex addict's blame-shifting and gaslighting tactics. Nobody should be subjected to inappropriate behaviour, be betrayed or lied to. However, after discovery or disclosure, you must bear full responsibility for what you allow and disallow moving forwards because you now know the addict's capabilities. As a result, clear boundaries are needed to keep you and everyone else well protected.

Impulsivity and compulsivity are the hallmarks of a sexual addiction. Sex addicts by nature act how they please, when they please, with no concern for the repercussions to their partner or for others. Throughout active recovery and healing, boundaries are the antidotes to compulsive sexual behaviours that indicate what behaviours are acceptable and what aren't. Recovering addicts and the betrayed partners must learn and adapt to these boundaries. Boundaries provide safety, room for change, healing, and restitution for the couple. In order to prevent re-traumatization, boundaries draw a clear line in the sand about what is appropriate for the individuals and their relationship. Defined boundaries also offer relationship regulation and self-protection. After a betrayal, there is usually always some ambiguity about what appropriate boundaries are and, more importantly, how to enforce them. Setting boundaries is a must and an act of self-compassion, according to Brené Brown (2010). Boundaries can be difficult and uncomfortable but are crucial first steps in regaining control over how you let your partner treat you rather than an attempt to control their addiction. These are the key components needed to reclaim confidence and take ownership of your life and actions.

A good boundary establishes the parameters of how the individuals will communicate and interact post betrayal. The betrayed partner must establish boundaries in order to express their needs and determine what is required for their safety in order to continue in the relationship.

Effective boundaries enable relationships to be strengthened and trust to be re-developed. The addict is more driven to take control of their actions, and others who support them may feel more comfortable offering assistance. There is less chance of enabling than of encouraging because any prospective support comes with boundaries and consequences. It takes time for the betrayed partner to establish boundaries after the betrayal. Being in a relationship with a recovering sex addict is difficult because they have many deeply embedded past behavioural patterns, which initially make it difficult to maintain boundaries. The betrayed partner needs to be aware of their own internal and external worries and learn how to effectively protect oneself by enforcing clear boundaries. After experiencing betrayal, you shouldn't compromise on what you require in order to feel safe and protected. The kind of boundaries required for present safety is determined by a combination of the safety issues encountered in the past and the predicted likelihood of similar concerns in the future. However, as the betrayed partners and their relationship evolve, boundaries may need to change for them.

The following are some examples of boundaries for a sex addict partner:

- No communication with the affair partners. Never at all.
- No more friendships with opposite gender.
- Absolutely no more flirting or sexualised language with others.
- Delete all unauthorised phone numbers, email addresses, applications, and dating websites.
- Computer browser histories can no longer be deleted.
- Complete disclosure and an end to all deception.
- Unfriend everyone you interacted with inappropriately on Facebook or other social media platforms.
- No more binge drinking.
- Giving up late-night internet browsing.
- To pass a polygraph test every 12 months to ensure sobriety.
- No more gambling or reckless spending.
- Installing pornographic filtering software on all of your devices.
- No relationships outside of our relationship, whether sexual or otherwise.
- No watching of porn or masturbating.
- Frequent sessions with the therapist.
- Attending 12-step program.
- Zero drug use.
- Educating yourself about SA and relationship restoration.
- No more gaslighting, manipulation or defensiveness.

How to set boundaries?
When setting boundaries, American Addiction Centres (2022) suggests that you consider these questions:

- Am I making time for myself to manage my stress?
- Am I establishing healthy boundaries for myself?

Each relationship will have a different set of boundaries because each one is unique. Your boundary might be, that your sex addict partner seeks treatment for their sex addiction, or they stop watching porn.

- **Consider the exact behaviour or behaviours for which you want to establish boundaries**

    Although you have no control over your partner's behaviour, your boundaries should make it obvious which behaviours you do and do not accept. Your boundary might, be that your partner's digital gadgets have a filter that prevents them from viewing porn. Or any lies or secrets must be revealed within a specific period of time.

- **Boundaries cannot be used as punishments.**

    Instead of inflicting pain to your addict partner while setting boundaries, be honest with yourself and think about safety as the main goal. A boundary cannot, for instance, mandate that the addict cuts all ties with their parents because they failed to support the betrayed partner after the reveal. Instead, restrictions should be placed on the circumstances and methods of interaction; for instance, the addict can still have relationships with them without involving the betrayed partner.

- **The boundary ought to promote individual accountability.**
  You might include conditions when setting a boundary that promote growth and more responsible behaviour. For instance, your boundary can be that the addict cannot move back home unless they stop lying or stonewalling and get counselling. The decision is then made by your addict partner, who now has control and responsibility over the results.

- **Set boundaries out of love and self-compassion.**
  Setting boundaries requires that you respond in a compassionate manner. The goal is not retaliation. Unless your addict partner wants to change, you cannot change them. Set boundaries based on the reality that the only person you can control is yourself. Your boundaries should be clear and indicate that you won't tolerate any continuous dysfunctional behaviour even though you love and respect your partner as well as value your own self-respect and self-compassion.

- **Boundaries must have a purpose**
  Additionally, when setting boundaries, it is important to gain an awareness of your needs and desires and learn how to fulfil them. Boundaries will remove any assumptions and clearly communicate how to approach the other partner in order to meet relationship needs. Most importantly, boundaries will allow you to figure out if your addict partner is able to gain your trust and respect by being dependable and accountable. Be aware to follow through with your own boundaries otherwise you allow the sex addict to continue hurting you. It is not

love to put up with your addict's reckless behaviour. Supporting their harmful behaviour against you or their cruel treatment of others is unacceptable.

Consequences for violation of a boundary

Consequences and boundaries are connected and cannot function apart. You define unacceptable behaviours and attitudes with boundaries, and you outline the steps you'll take if these boundaries are breached. Creating boundaries alone is insufficient without ability to employ them. What happens, though, when a line is crossed and an important boundary pertaining to a behavioural standard is violated? How does this situation relate to a consequence? What precise consequence is appropriate in this situation, and how may it be carried out? Once the addict partner is aware that their actions could result in consequences, they can choose whether or not they are willing to accept the possibility of having to face that consequence. Often I encounter that when couples recognise and set the needed boundaries, they frequently fail to respect them. Their failure to take into account the crucial components of the boundary core issue led to this. Personal boundaries without consequences are not even remotely effective or protective. Consequences are the results of someone's actions and we all know that sex addiction is about engagement in out of control and risky sexual conducts without any regards to consequences for self and others. A consequence is what happens as a result of an action. The word outcome or consequence comes from the Latin sequ, which also means to lead or precede (Nichol, 2007). There are several definitions that all give similar meanings:

1. Anything that is brought about by a cause.

2. An outcome of activities, especially if that outcome is unwelcome or disagreeable.

3. A proposition derived from the agreement of several prior propositions; an inference; any conclusion reached by reasoning or argument.

4. It is a cause-and-effect relationship.

5. Importance in relation to what.

6. The capacity to exert influence or cause a reaction.

Consequences might be either positive or negative. **Positive consequences** reinforce behaviour and increase the likelihood that it will occur again. Positive feedback, appreciation, and incentives for good behaviour are examples of positive consequences. You can restart date nights, for instance, if your addict partner regularly attends individual and couple therapy sessions and uses the tools they acquire to promote relational safety. When there are **negative consequences**, behaviour is less likely to happen again. There are some circumstances in which you might choose to use strict consequences for your addict partner's inappropriate sexual behaviour. For instance, if they continue to view porn or masturbate, the result is that they must leave the house for a predetermined period of time.

When discussing self-control, personal or relational safety, the phrases consequence and punishment are frequently confused. Consequences and punishments are two different concepts with two different purposes.

What are boundaries

Punishment is the act of harming someone physically or mentally. You may use punishments that are motivated by anger and fear, meant to inflict shame, and frequently appear to be a withholding of affection in order to get someone to do as you ask. In addition, the desire for control and emotional drive are what lead to the imposition of punishments.

In the early stages following discovery and disclosure, when the betrayed partner has likely felt extremely defenceless, powerless, and emotionally scarred, punishment often provides a sense of pain alleviation and control. Punishment, however, is certainly the most harmful and sometimes addictive behaviour that betrayed partners can engage in. Please stop shaming and punishing your addict partner if you are. Why? Because punishment might prolong the pain you are trying so hard to relieve by slowing your healing and his sobriety processes. Continuously punishing, humiliating, or being spiteful will also be toxic to you and detrimental for your emotional and physical health. Moreover, both pleasant and unpleasant aspects of life are expressed in the existence and universe. There is a positive and negative duality to everything in the world. Nothing is absolutely either good or evil. This indicates that there are negative aspects to everyone and everything. Nevertheless, every drawback has a plus side as well. The two do not contradict one another. Your partner's addiction may not have been the only negative aspect of him. Maybe you could focus on some of his positive qualities. I am aware that this is a difficult task in the wake of the traumatising betrayal but attempt to identify any gains or benefits following the discovery and disclosure. This will assist you in taming the punisher inside who wants to inflict the suffering that the sex addict caused. Instead of being a perfectionist and expecting your addict partner to move from 0 to 100 overnight, put your focus on and appreciate their small successes. The fact is that they simply are unable to complete the recovery process at the speed you desire or even deserve. It is what it is. After all, they are only human. Instead of perfection, pay attention to progress. If you chose option B, separation, keep your attention on your strengths and abilities as you navigate this difficult route. Regardless of the current state of your relationship with the addict, learn to love and accept progress over perfection. I have occasionally seen betrayed partners who are uncomfortable attending group therapy or workshops because they believe other couples have done much better or other betrayed partners are healing more quickly. While they still exist in the cycle of pain, bitterness and punishment of their addict partner. The unease you the betrayed partner experience when you witness other betrayed partners being more content, confident, expressive, grieving openly, telling their truth without shame, making progress and loving themselves is genuine. However, you don't resent those individuals or want them to be smaller. This is simply a crystal-clear sign of what you must do in order to heal, un-stuck yourself and end the punishment.

In summary punishment can create bitterness and resentment in both partners. Resentment or bitterness are like stabbing yourself but expecting the other person to feel the pain. Furthermore, the amount of recovery efforts must increase in direct proportion to the severity of the imposed punishment . The challenges that already exist in a relationship are made worse by punishment. As a result, additional repairs are required because the restoration needs are growing and taking longer. There is no question that because of the compulsive and deceptive sexual behaviours of their mate, the betrayed partner experiences true, severe, and pervasive pain and suffering. However, trying to minimise pain on one side while simultaneously adding more through punishment is simply impossible. As long as something is being purposefully damaged, trying to fix it is challenging if not impossible. Because of the way our brains are designed, punishing another person emotionally rarely relieves our own pain or makes them want to connect to us.

What are boundaries

Contrary, consequences are used to protect safety, assume responsibility, and inform. The effects of one's actions are known as consequences. Your addict partner will learn from consequences that their actions are their own free will and obligation. You have the right to set the boundaries and the associated consequences when dealing with your sex addict partner. You get to select what is appropriate and what you will permit as a result of your partner's behavioural decisions. The desired boundaries and consequences must be fair and be largely constant once made and adequately conveyed to ensure that all parties are aware of the implications. Your expectations must be clear and understood by both of you. Therefore, it is crucial to draught an agreed-upon relationship or covenant contract that outlines all the boundaries and consequences in detail. The best outcome is attained when even the sex addict partner is encouraged to set personal and interpersonal boundaries for themselves that ensure everyone's safety. In addition, they may be asked to nominate their own consequences in the event that any boundary is broken and not respected or remedied within the predetermined time range. In this manner, the addict is once more taught to accept responsibility for their own actions and their outcomes.

Examples of consequences linked to established boundaries:

- Not allowed to sleep in the same bed.
- No sexual intimacy for ……..days.
- Reaching out to some men in 12- step group and admit to them your violation, gather the learnings and journal about them.
- Write an apology/repair letter, and an action plan and deliver it within 2 hours of a boundary violation.

- Cleaning the garage, house etc for 4 hours.
- Booking an urgent therapy session.
- No access to your phone for ....days.
- No smoking for ....days.
- Donating money to a cause or church that you dislike.
- Three months separation with limited contacts.
- Three months separation with zero contact.
- Permanent separation.

Your partner's addiction and his unhealthy behavioural patterns did not emerge suddenly. These are the results of years of ingrained behaviours and faulty coping mechanisms that need to be recognised, discussed and examined by both of you and your therapist. You can explain your perspectives, wants and needs, the justifications for your nominated boundaries, and the consequences for when you know that the relationship contract has been violated. This makes it simpler for you to communicate your values and how important they are for re-establishing your relationship with your recovering an addict partner.

The last step and undoubtedly the hardest for you is to separate from your addict partner's behaviours and let them drive their own boundary and consequence bus.

Once you've established boundaries, expressed them, and discussed the consequences, make sure you step back from your partner's decisions and behaviours. Keep in mind that only your own actions—not his—are within your control. Your boundaries are imposed, and depending on your partner's actions and consistency, they decide whether or not they want to be in a relationship with you. If they consistently violate your boundaries and refuse to make

What are boundaries

the relationship safe, you must take the necessary precautions to ensure your own safety.

Your boundaries are your safety and 100% your responsibility.

The challenges in maintaining boundaries and consequences, according to one betrayed partner:

One of my non-negotiable boundaries in our relationship contract was that my recovering husband stop watching porn. If he did, I proposed that our relationship would end with at least a 3 month separation. A violation of this boundary was detected by the polygraph test conducted later. After hours of therapy, my husband reluctantly admitted that he had relapsed and had used Etsy to view pornography. I had no idea that Etsy offered the ability to see porn. What in the world is going on? For a full year, he has worked so well. I moved the polygraph test forward because I could actually see the pattern of dishonesty, deception, and severe defensiveness this time more clearly. I had intended to leave for a few days later in order to maximise my confidence and find the strength to enforce my own boundaries and his consequence. But I was having trouble. Why was this so challenging? Did he know that he could easily violate my boundaries and that I wouldn't be able to hold him accountable? Am I enabling him?

Being alone with two young children was incredibly difficult. Was he using this information for his benefit? I had absolutely no idea what to do. I was unable to get out of bed. I knew I shouldn't have included that in our contract if I wasn't going to honour it following the relapse. Although I was in excruciating pain and questioned my abilities, I knew that the moment I didn't enforce my boundary, I was giving him permission to relapse and violate us once more. Instead of leaving, I asked him to leave right away while I went over what I was prepared to accept and what I was not. After making sure that I was honouring my own boundaries, which protected my family—including my children and his sobriety—I then validated myself and my decision. Having some crisis therapy during this time was absolutely invaluable for me to reaffirm that what I was doing was the right thing. However, being by myself, caring for two children and everything else while I was exhausted was terribly difficult. I had to keep in mind, though, that he had already made a choice for all of us, and there was nothing I could do but look out for myself. We created a formal separation agreement with boundaries with the aid of our therapist. He had to demonstrate that he had remained sober and had made progress towards recovery if he wished to return after three months. If he failed the polygraph test at the end of this period my clear boundary was a permanent separation, then. I have to admit that the first three months although challenging they were valuable to me since they pushed me to evaluate my own capabilities and give me a newfound confidence in the event that he wasn't able to maintain sobriety. I'm not letting him cross my boundaries anymore, and I'm not afraid to quit if and when he puts his addiction before his family. Today marks nine months of steady sobriety and the restoration of our relationships. But I refuse to live in fear of the future since I now know what my boundaries are, and even if he crosses them in 20 years, I won't be scared to take the necessary measures to safeguard my safety, values, and dignity.

As for Etsy, I have looked further into it and you can find anything on Etsy, Pinterest, Tumblr, Facebook, Instagram etc. These are often sites that men use to find porn because it can fly under the radar.

Anita, wife of a sex addict.

CHAPTER 13

Holistic treatment plan based on betrayal trauma model

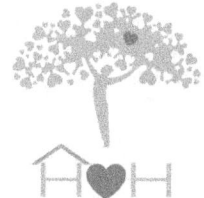

Can trauma from betrayal be treated?

To this, there is no simple solution. Reminding ourselves once more that trauma is a subjective experience, each person has different needs when trying to cope with it. After the discovery or disclosure day, it could take months for some people while it might take years for others before they feel they are out of the woods.

Even years later, trauma reactions can still happen. They might not be full- blown and out of control, but if you don't focus on your recovery and use your skills, they might still be.

According to my academic and clinical experiences, recovery from betrayal trauma requires intentionality and a holistic approach. Due to the complexity of this multidimensional trauma, there can never be a single toll that can address all of its facets.

Following are a few holistic strategies that can aid the betrayed partner in their healing process:

- Individual and relational therapy
- Trauma therapy
- Talk therapy
- Relational Boundary setting
- Feeling journaling
- EMDR
- Neuro feedback
- Group therapy
- Meditation
- Yoga
- Physical exercise
- Gratitude journaling
- Art therapy
- Medication

The betrayed partner must take certain actions to ensure that the healing process moves forwards without becoming stalled in the grief and pain cycles.

1. Educate yourself about sex addiction and betrayal trauma

Despite the fact that sex addiction is never about the betrayed partner, they frequently take it personally and assume they must be lacking in some way for their partners to engage in compulsive sexual behaviours. Such notions make them wonder if they are desirable, attractive, or good enough. These misconceptions are all common emotional reactions that can be somewhat addressed by becoming more knowledgeable about addictions. My suggestion is that you will experience more comfort as you gain knowledge about addiction, including how your partner got caught up in it, how it affects their brains, and how they will require support to recover. When you acknowledge that this is the beast of all addictions and has nothing to do with you, you may reclaim your freedom and hope.

2. The betrayed partner shouldn't isolate or blame themselves

It's normal to feel betrayed and duped after learning about your partner's addiction and to believe that your partner intentionally hurt your feelings. Alternately, you can feel false guilt and believe that their actions are somehow your fault. Pain from trauma drives you to create a wall around yourself. It's normal to feel the want to retreat from your addict partner, other people, and situations, but it's crucial to fight this impulse. Create a network of supportive individuals around you, attend therapy, seek comfort in a safe community, and learn to speak openly and honestly with trustworthy people. The truth is that, however unintended your partner's actions have inflicted excruciating pain and made you doubt not only your relationships but also your own beliefs and values. Furthermore, blaming yourself for your partner's addiction will only make it harder for you to support and care for yourself. Though it might be challenging, try to constantly remind yourself that nobody else's actions are your responsibility.

3. Learn about the signs of your own trauma

Betrayal trauma brought on by sex addiction is one of the most complex traumas to recover from since it shatters your sense of self and makes you wonder who you can trust. It's simple to get caught up in a cycle of dread, uncertainties, hopelessness, rage, anxiety, and controlling behaviours when you're experiencing pain and grief from betrayal. Recognize your trauma responses, which may include disordered eating habits, detective behaviours, pessimistic views of others, self-harm or suicidal thoughts, or the need to isolate yourself. As soon as you can, seek expert assistance and learn how to manage some of your own symptoms. Additionally, it's critical that you establish self-regulation and self-care routines.

4. Develop a personalised daily recovery schedule

Create a customised daily recovery planner with the assistance of your therapist. If you've chosen to stay in a relationship with a recovering sex addict, your schedule must include relational and individual recovery work. Create time each day to reflect on your established boundaries and consequences, write in a journal about your feelings and triggers, engage in some creative activities, go for a walk or a meditation session, dance to music, go swimming, practise yoga, or do anything else that helps you feel like you've taken care of yourself. Simply taking yourself out for coffee or ice cream is all you need to do at times. Have daily pre-scheduled times where you and your partner can share your emotions, difficulties, and gratitude to one another. Communication is crucial if you want to mend the connection. Share your aspirations with one another and engage in enjoyable activities. Each of you needs a self-care regimen that satisfies your unique emotional needs.

5. Find a good specialist therapist for your individual and relationship restoration

Therapy for sexual addiction is crucial, and betrayed partners frequently feel compelled to attend counselling. They frequently question me *why do I have to do all of this work since he was the one who perpetrated all of these heinous acts? Why isn't he able to come here by himself, complete the necessary work, and fix himself?*

I always give the same answer when someone asks me this question: both of you need relational therapy to learn how to interact to one another and establish intimacy, even while he needs individual therapy, and you need it to deal with the trauma of your betrayal. Sex addiction is, after all, an interpersonal incapability or intimacy dysfunction that must be treated in the context of the relationship. Additionally, while going through the continuing healing process, the betrayed partner needs to learn how to create boundaries and protect themselves. Which all need to be discussed, agreed upon, and learned in therapy. At the end of the first session, however, I frequently observe that the majority of the same betrayed partners who initially on their phone interview resisted coming in acknowledge the value of both individual and couple therapy and express gratitude for the knowledge and empowerment they have acquired.

6. Support your recovering sex addict partner while avoiding fixing or enabling them

Try not to punish or sabotage your partner if you want to keep your relationship together. Although it will take some time, make every effort to assist yourself and your partner in the rebuilding process. Rebuilding trust is a process that never ends in recovery so seek safety in the meantime. Be patient with yourself and keep in mind that your partner is also recovering from a severe addiction. Furthermore, quit even attempting to change, fix or save your partner because you have no control over their actions! You cannot force your partner to change, no matter how hard you try. Your sex addict partner is the only one who is actually capable of changing their behaviour and dismantling their behavioural patterns.

Nevertheless, supporting your partner and allowing them to maintain their addiction are quite different things. Make your partner aware of your love and support for them, but also work on developing healthy boundaries that will help them acknowledge and address their addiction. If your partner relapses or makes deliberate indiscretions, it's crucial to forgive them and avoid shaming them; nevertheless, doing so while trying to minimize what happened or protect them from the consequences is enabling them. Therefore, they may find it more difficult to break the habit. As a betrayed partner, don't be responsible for keeping your partner sober. Avoid getting too involved in controlling or watching over your partner's compulsive sexual behaviour. Instead the sex addict must take responsibility for their own self-evaluation. Otherwise, toxic co-dependency that is detrimental to recovery will develop.

7. Avoid sexual intimacy with your addict partner until you are certain they are STD-free and have stopped engaging in any risky sexual behaviours

Betrayed partners shouldn't feel pressured to engage in sexual activities with their partners until the sex addict partners have restored their safety and trust. Given that sex addicts may infect their partners with STDs (Sexually Transmitted Diseases), having safe sex or complete abstinence may be essential. Up until the betrayed partners are prepared to resume sexual intimacy, the recovering sex addict can find other healthy alternatives to sexual connection, such as meditation, exercise, 12-step meetings, reaching out to a sponsor, etc.

8. Accept your emotions instead of avoiding them

A variety of negative emotions may manifest following a betrayal. It's common to feel inferior or humiliated. The feelings of fury, vengeance, sickness, and grief are also possible. Naturally, in an effort to avoid this discomfort, you might find yourself attempting to avoid or block what happened which can make it more challenging to manage them. You need to accept what happened and address the accompanying feelings before you can begin to heal. If you don't deal with the difficult feelings when they arise, your anxiety may spread to other aspects of your life. No matter how hard you try to suppress or ignore them, you can still have triggers or thoughts related to them when you're at work, with relatives or taking care of your kids. It can be simpler and less terrifying to sit with those emotions and gradually raise your awareness of them. Once you have a better knowledge of your feelings, you may devise strategies for handling them more skilfully. Leaning into challenging emotions could be too difficult to even consider after a trauma like betrayal. Accepting negative emotions, enables you to begin investigating the causes and potential solutions, which in turn could promote the healing process.

9. Take care of your financial health

Having financial stability is crucial for betrayal partners during recovering. A common reason why a betrayed partner maintains an unhealthy relationship with a sex addict who can't seem to stop indulging in his compulsive or destructive behaviours is a lack of financial independence. You will approach this journey differently than someone without resources if you can manage to have some sort of financial means, whether it comes from your own employment, a business, an investment, or the knowledge that you could obtain financial security through a divorce. You will have an additional challenge if you are going through this process without any real income, retirement assets, or savings. If you believe you lack the skills or resources to support yourself independently from your addict partner, you will feel less empowered and approach the healing from betrayal trauma, reconciliation, or even separation differently than someone with stable finances. I urge you to start working on your independence and enhancing your financial fitness so that you won't feel compelled to put up with the abuse of sex addiction.

10. Establish a safe space for mindfulness and self-regulation exercises

A safe place is a calm, cosy setting where you can withdraw mentally during trying moments. Having many safe spaces is advantageous. Some examples include a special room in the house, a hideaway corner with some comfy pillows and fluffy objects, a garden, a convenient park or beach. When needing to retreat to your safe space use five senses to self-regulate. The more senses you use to describe your safe place, the better. Develop a mindfulness practise in your safe space as well by being totally present in every moment without passing judgement or criticism. When you are mindful, you pay attention to everything going on around you rather than dozing off or becoming lost in your own thoughts about the past or the future. When you feel yourself being overtaken by negative emotions, mindfulness can help you regain your equilibrium so that you are not ruled by them.

11. When triggered or having a trauma response, use self-regulation/ self-soothing or opposite action techniques

Some of the many types of health self-soothing practises to explore is five senses or sensory soothing, opposite actions and fact checking.

Five senses or sensory soothing- is a simple but very effective approach to achieve self-regulation. This can be done using the five senses (*sight, hearing, taste, smell*, and *touch*). All you have to do is be present, focus on your senses, and let yourself be completely absorbed in the sensory experience. This is how it's done:

Step 1 - Take 5 deep breaths in and out.
Step 2 - Name 4 items you see.
Step 3 - Name 3 objects you can touch.
Step 4 - Name 2 things you hear.
Step 5 - Name 1 thing you can smell.

Self-soothing or self-regulation examples:

1) Focus on your breathing.
2) Change your environment.
3) Stretch and move your body.
4) Journaling.
5) Engage in a creative activity such as painting, dancing or playing an instrument.
6) Play a game of chess.
7) Take a shower or bath.
8) Tranquil imagery. Such as a burning candle, soft lighting, photographs of loved ones, affirmations etc.
9) Relaxing music.
10) Practice self-love and self-compassion by Speaking kindly and lovingly to yourself aloud.
11) Mindful walking.
12) Meditation.
13) Practice 5 senses or sensory soothing.

How to self-regulate/self-soothe

1-There is a triggering event, feeling, or thinking (i.e., something happens that provokes a reaction, or a negative emotion).

2-You take a breath, pay attention, notice and identify what is going on, both cognitively (understanding it) and emotionally (feeling it), but you decide to try other coping mechanisms.

3-You select appropriate coping strategies (e.g., sitting in emotions, praying, journaling, connecting with others, therapy, and so on).

Holistic treatment plan based on betrayal trauma model

This is what you do to control and regulate your feelings about the trigger or the activities you take to address it.

4-When emotional dysregulation caused you to have angry outbursts in the past, your healthy coping skills now will have the opposite and more favourable outcomes.

5-By utilising positive self-soothing techniques you're assisting your own brain in shifting control away from the limbic system and towards the prefrontal cortex for more executive decision-making. Consequently, your brain will begin to rewire itself and become accustomed to the new pattern of self-soothing and self-control if you employ the same healthy self-regulating methods repeatedly. In contrast, if you continue to give in and engage in unhealthy self-soothing behaviours (withdrawal or rage), you will just reinforce your brain's previous programming and enhance the responsiveness of the limbic system.

Opposite action and check the facts when triggered- Use this technique when you are triggered, have an intrusive thought, or you experience a specific negative emotion, which is usually followed by a specific behaviour depending on that emotion. For example, you may believe your partner has disrespected you (thought) by not protecting their eyes, become enraged (feeling), and fight (behaviour) with them, or the thought may make you sad, causing you to withdraw yourself from others. Ultimately, your body causes you to react to your thoughts and emotions in a certain way. Engaging in opposite actions means challenging the initial negative or unpleasant thought. Assess the truthfulness of that thought. Is it based on feelings or facts? Having a thought does not always imply that it is real. To help minimise the strength of these intense emotions, check the facts in the moment. Choose to examine the facts to assist you to change your emotional response and make healthier decisions as a result of unpleasant emotions. You can adjust your response to a level suitable for the situation or respond with a more appropriate attitude by using check the facts and doing the opposite actions.

Ask yourself:

- *Do the facts justify the intensity of my emotional responses?*
- *What can I do that is the total opposite of my usual reaction?*

For example, instead of yelling when you're angry, consider speaking quietly and respectfully.

It is therapeutic and healing to share your story among trusted people

Sharing your story with others often helps you to process it at a deeper and healthier level. This can happen in a setting that is secure and supportive, such as group therapy or with a close friend or therapist with whom you have developed a relationship. It's crucial to have the capacity to communicate one's authentic self. Your chances of recovering are higher if you learn to share your truth with the support of encouraging people. In addition to trying to make sense of the significant betrayals that have irreversibly altered their lives, a betrayed partner may come off as nuts since they have probably spent years being deceived, manipulated, and given the blame for everything by their addict partner. Everyone must first realise that trauma isn't about trying to con or control other people or about playing games. Trauma is NEVER a choice rather it is the psychological consequence of a strong, ingrained conviction that you are inherently unsafe. Trauma and being traumatised are about survival, not about arguing a point. Betrayal trauma is sometimes an ill-defined and misunderstood condition, but when it receives the appropriate attention for healing, it may pave the

Holistic treatment plan based on betrayal trauma model

way for growth, enlightenment and advancement on the spiritual path. You are free to choose the best healing route for you. Then by all means, go ahead and share your story and select the optimum healing you are entitled to because you matter and are more capable than you may realise.

References

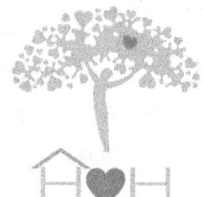

1. Allen, E. S., & Atkins, D. C. (2012). The Association of Divorce and Extramarital Sex in a Representative U.S. Sample. Journal of Family Issues, 33(11), 1477–1493. https://doi.org/10.1177/0192513x12439692

2. Allen, E. S., Atkins, D. C., Baucom, D. H., Snyder, D. K., Gordon, K. C., & Glass, S. P. (2006). Intrapersonal, Interpersonal, And Contextual Factors in Engaging in and Responding to Extramarital Involvement. Clinical Psychology: Science and Practice, 12(2), 101–130. https://doi.org/10.1093/clipsy.bpi014

3. American Addiction Centers. (2022). Signs of Codependency & Addiction. https://americanaddictioncenters.org/rehab-guide/codependent-relationship

4. American Psychiatric Association (APA). (2013). Diagnostic and statistical manual of mental disorders (DSM-5®). American Psychiatric Pub.

5. American Society of Addiction Medicine (ASAM). (2011). Public Policy Statement: Definition of Addiction. https://www.asam.

org/docs/default-source/public-policy-statements/1definition_of_addiction_long_4-11.pdf?sfvrsn=a8f64512_4#:~:text=Addiction%20is%20a%20primary%2C%20chronic,psychological%2C%20social%20and%20spiritual%20manifestations

6. Anderson, P. B., & Morgan, M. (1994). Spirituality and sexuality: The healthy connection. Journal of Religion and Health, 33(2), 115–121. https://doi.org/10.1007/bf02354531

7. Andrade, C. (2020). The limitations of online surveys. Indian Journal of Psychological Medicine, 42(6), 575-576. https://doi.org/10.1177/0253717620957496

8. Andrews, T. (2012). What is Social Constructism? The Grounded Theory Review, 11(1), 39–46. http://groundedtheoryreview.com/2012/06/01/what-is-social-constructionism

9. Antevska, A., & Gavey, N. (2015). 'Out of Sight and Out of Mind': Detachment and men's consumption of male sexual dominance and female submission in pornography. Men and Masculinities, 18(5), 605–629. https://doi.org/10.1177/1097184x15574339

10. Banz, B. C., Yip, S. W., Yau, Y. H., & Potenza, M. N. (2016). Behavioural addictions in addiction medicine. Progress in Brain Research, 223, 311–328. https://doi.org/10.1016/bs.pbr.2015.08.003

11. Barna Group. (2016). The Porn Phenomenon: The impact of pornography. https://www.barna.com/the-porn-phenomenon/

12. Barth, R. J., & Kinder, B. N. (1987). The mislabeling of sexual impulsivity. Journal of Sex & Marital Therapy, 13(1), 15–23. https://doi.org/10.1080/00926238708403875

13. Baumeister, R. F., & Leary, M. R. (1995). The need to belong: Desire for interpersonal attachments as a fundamental human motivation. Psychological Bulletin, 117(3), 497–529. https://doi.org/10.1037/0033-2909.117.3.497

14. Becker, C. S. (1992). Living and Relating: An Introduction to Phenomenolgy. Sage.

References

15. Becker, L. (2018). Methodological proposals for the study of consumer experience. Qualitative Market Research: An International Journal, 21(4), 465–490. https://doi.org/10.1108/qmr-01-2017-0036

16. Beltrán-Morillas, A. M., Valor-Segura, I., & Expósito, F. (2019). Unforgiveness Motivations in Romantic Relationships Experiencing Infidelity: Negative Affect and Anxious Attachment to the Partner as Predictors. Frontiers in Psychology, 10. https://doi.org/10.3389/fpsyg.2019.00434

17. Bendt, P. (2020). Self-gaslighting in Sexual Assault: A feminist approach to reclaiming agency. Johns Hopkins University.

18. Birchard, T., & Benfield, J. (2017). Routledge international handbook of sexual addiction. Routledge.

19. Black, C. (2019). Deceived: Facing the trauma of sexual betrayal. Central Recovery Press.

20. Black, C., & Tripodi, C. (2012). Intimate treason: Healing the trauma for partners confronting sex addiction. Central Recovery Press.

21. Black, D. W., Kehrberg, L. L., Flumerfelt, D. L., & Schlosser, S. S. (1997). Characteristics of 36 subjects reporting compulsive sexual behaviour. The American Journal of Psychiatry, 154(2), 243–249. https://www.ncbi.nlm.nih.gov/pubmed/9016275

22. Bliss, L. A. (2016). Phenomenological research. International Journal of Adult Vocational Education and Technology, 7(3), 14–26. https://doi.org/10.4018/ijavet.2016070102

23. Bloomberg, L. D., & Volpe, M. (2016). Completing Your Qualitative Dissertation: a Road Map from Beginning to End (3rd ed.). Sage.

24. Böthe, B., Koós, M., Tóth-Király, I., Orosz, G., & Demetrovics, Z. (2019). Investigating the Associations of Adult ADHD Symptoms, Hypersexuality, and Problematic Pornography Use Among Men and Women on a Largescale, Non-Clinical Sample. *The Journal of Sexual Medicine*, 16(4), 489–499. https://doi.org/10.1016/j.jsxm.2019.01.312

25. Böthe, B., Potenza, M. N., Griffiths, M. D., Kraus, S. W., Klein, V., Fuss, J., & Demetrovics, Z. (2020). The development

of the Compulsive Sexual Behaviour Disorder Scale (CSBD-19): An ICD-11 based screening measure across three languages. Journal of Behavioural Addictions, 9(2), 247–258. https://doi.org/10.1556/2006.2020.00034

26. Bowcott, O. (2014). Lie Detector Tests Begin on Sex Offenders. The Guardian.

27. Bowen, M. (1985). Family therapy in clinical practice. Jason Aronson.

28. Bowlby, J. (1969). *Attachment and loss: Attachment*. Basic Books.

29. Bowlby, J. (1977). The Making and Breaking of Affectional Bonds. British Journal of Psychiatry, 130(3), 201–210. https://doi.org/10.1192/bjp.130.3.201

30. Bowlby, J. (1982). Attachment and Loss. Basic Books. http://changingminds.org/explanations/trust/what_is_trust.htm

31. Boyle, J. S. (1991). Field research: A collaborative model for practice and research. Qualitative Nursing Research: A Contemporary Dialogue, 273–299. https://doi.org/10.4135/9781483349015.n32

32. Bożek, A., Nowak, P. F., & Blukacz, M. (2020). The Relationship Between Spirituality, Health-Related Behaviour, and Psychological Wellbeing. Frontiers in Psychology, 11(1997). https://doi.org/10.3389/fpsyg.2020.01997

33. Braun-Harvey, D., & Vigorito, M. A. (2016). Treating out of control sexual behaviour: rethinking sex addiction. Springer.

34. Braun, V., & Clarke, V. (2006). Using thematic analysis in psychology. Qualitative Research in Psychology, 3(2), 77–101. https://doi.org/10.1191/1478088706qp063oa

35. Braun, V., Clarke, V., & Gray, D. (2017). Collecting qualitative data: A practical guide to textual, media and virtual techniques. Cambridge University Press.

36. Braun, V., Clarke, V., & Hayfield, N. (2019). 'A starting point for your journey, not a map': Nikki Hayfield in conversation with Virginia Braun and Victoria Clarke about thematic analysis. Qualitative

References

Research in Psychology, 19(2), 1–22. https://doi.org/10.1080/14780887.2019.1670765

37. Briere, J. N., & Scott, C. (2015). Principles of trauma therapy: A guide to symptoms, evaluation, and treatment (DSM-5 update). Sage.

38. Brown, B. (2010). The gifts of imperfection: Let go of who you think you're supposed to be and embrace who you are. Simon and Schuster.

39. Bryman, A. (2016). Social Research Methods. Oxford University Press.

40. Burr, V. (2015). Social Constructionism. Routledge.

41. Büssing, A., Baumann, K., Hvidt, N. C., Koenig, H. G., Puchalski, C. M., & Swinton, J. (2014). Spirituality and health. Evidence-Based Complementary and Alternative Medicine, 2014, 1–2. https://doi.org/10.1155/2014/682817

42. Carnes, P. (1991). Don't call it love: Recovery from sexual addiction. Bantam Books.

43. Carnes, P. (2000). Sexual Addiction and Complusion: Recognition, Treatment and Recover. CNS Spectrums, 5(10), 63–74. https://doi.org/10.1017/s1092852900007689

44. Carnes, P. (2009). Out of the shadows: Understanding sexual addiction. Simon & Schuster.

45. Carnes, P. (2011). Recovery Start Kit: A 100-day plan for addiction recovery. Gentle Path Press.

46. Carnes, P. (2013). Don't call it love: Recovery from sexual addiction. Bantam.

47. Carnes, P. (2015). The Whole and the Sum of the Parts … Towards a More Inclusive Understanding of Divergences in Sexual Behaviours. Sexual Addiction & Compulsivity, 22(2), 105–108. https://doi.org/10.1080/10720162.2015.1050329

48. Carnes, P. (2018). Betrayal Bond, Revised: Breaking Free of Exploitive Relationships. HCI.

49. Carnes, P. J. (2019). The Sexual Addiction Screening Process. Clinical Management of Sex Addiction, 21-39. https://doi.org/10.4324/9781315755267-4

50. Carnes, P., & Adams, K. M. (2013). Clinical management of sex addiction. Routledge

51. Corley, M. D., & Hook, J. N. (2012). Women, Female and Sex and Love Addicts, and Use of the Internet. *Sexual Addiction & Compulsivity, 19*(1-2), 53-76. https://doi.org/10.1080/10720162.2012.660430

52. Fawcett, D. (2022). *Approval-Seeking Behaviour.* https://sexandrelationshiphealing.com/blog/approval-seeking-behavior/

53. https://www.thesun.co.uk/news/2412759/dogging-sites-public-sex-illegal-uk-where/

54. Manning, J. (2022). *Polygraph Testing in sex Addiction Recover: A Foothold for Rebuilding Trust, Affirming 'Gut' & Fostering Accountability.* https://drjillmanning.com/polygraph-testing-in-sex-addiction-recovery/

55. Meijer, E. H., & van Koppen, P. J. (2017). Lie detectors and the law: The use of the polygraph in Europe. In *Psychology and law* (pp. 45-64). Routledge.

56. Nichol, M. (2007). *Words That Follow "Sequi".* https://www.dailywritingtips.com/words-that-follow-sequi/

57. Saldžiunas, V., & Kovalenko, A. (2008). The Event Knowledge Test (EKT). *POLYGRAPH.* https://repozytorium.ka.edu.pl/bitstream/handle/11315/801/Eurpoean_Polygraph_nr1_2008.pdf?sequence=6#page=21

58. Stevenson, A. (Ed.). (2010). *Oxford dictionary of English.* Oxford University Press, USA.

59. Vaughan, P. (2003). *The Monogamy Myth: A Personal Handbook for Recovering.* Newmarket Press.

60. Vaughan, P. (2003). *The monogamy myth: A personal handbook for recovering from affairs.* William Morrow Paperbacks.

61. Weiss. (2020). Characteristics of *Intimacy Anorexia.* https://intimacyanorexia.com/intimacy-anorexia-characteristics-2/

About Author

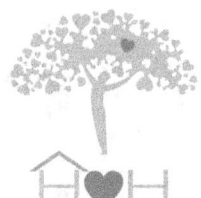

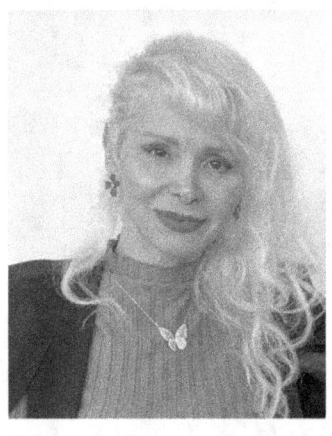

Dr Fai Seyed lives in Brisbane, Australia, and has a PhD in sex addiction and its impact on female partners' well-being and lived experiences. In addition, she has a master's degree in counselling and psychotherapy, is a supervisor and trainer, and is a qualified oral and dental surgeon from Sweden. She has over 27 years of clinical experience in both public and private practice across Sweden, England, and Australia.

Dr Fai is an accomplished author of multiple books and academic articles on sex addiction and betrayal trauma in partners. Interacting with patients, friends, family members, staff, and other stakeholders who have struggled with sexual addiction has motivated her to progress in this field. Dr Seyed is working with sexual addicts and their partners and has designed a unique structured 12-week recovery and reconciliation framework.

Qualifications:
PhD, Master of counselling, Clinical counsellor/Supervisor SRT (Sexual Recovery therapist), Partners Betrayal Trauma therapy, Gottman (L1, L2), TRTP practitioner
Neurofeedback provider, Sex addiction therapist, AASAT (American association of sex addiction therapy),
ACA level 3, CCAA reg. PACFA (Clinical)
(Dental/Oral surgeon BDS, Sweden)

www.houseofhopecounselling.com.au

enquiries@houseofhopecounselling.com.au

Services and Offers

Sex addiction therapy for individuals and their partners (AASAT; American Association for Sex Addiction Therapy), AASAT Betrayal Partner Recovery Specialist, AASAT Intimacy Anorexia Specialist, Gottman (level 1, 2), NLP, Hypnosis, NeurOptimal® neurofeedback, EMDR, trauma and PTSD management, infidelity recovery, Gestalt therapy, cognitive behavioural therapy, mindfulness practice, betrayal trauma, ADHD, depression and family therapy.

Bonus for finishing this book:
30 minutes free consultation with Dr Fai where you can have all your questions answered in private.

Contact details
Ph. 0413 482 486

www.houseofhopecounsellingcentre.com.au
enquiries@houseofhopecounselling.com.au

Peer reviewed Publications

Seyed Aghamiri, F. & Luetz, J.M. (2021). Sexual addiction and Christian education—An emerging research agenda. In J. M. Luetz & B. Green (Eds.), Innovating Christian education research—Multidisciplinary perspectives (pp. 443–468). Springer Nature. https://doi.org/10.1007/978-981-15-8856-3_24

Seyed Aghamiri, F., Luetz, J. M., & Hills, K. (2022). Innovating Research on Compulsive Sexual Behaviours. [Under peer review]

Seyed Aghamiri, F., Luetz, J. M., & Hills, K. (2022). Impacts of Sexual Addiction on Intimate Female Partners—The State of the Art, Sexual Health & Compulsivity, https://doi.org/10.1080/26929953.2022.2050862

Seyed Aghamiri, F., Luetz, J. M., Hills, K. (2022). Pornography addiction and its impacts on intimate female partner wellbeing—A systematic narrative synthesis. Journal of Addictive Diseases. https://doi.org/10550887.2021.2021058

The Long-Lived Impacts of Sexual Addiction: Examples of Unwanted Gifts That Keep Giving Fakri Seyed Aghamiro & Johannes M. Luetz https://doi.org/10.1080/26929953.2022.2163013

Other books by Dr Fai Seyed

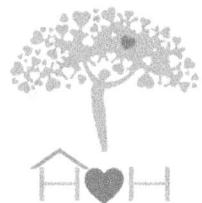

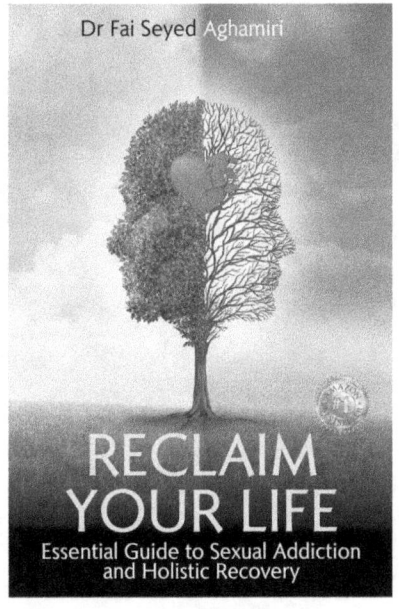

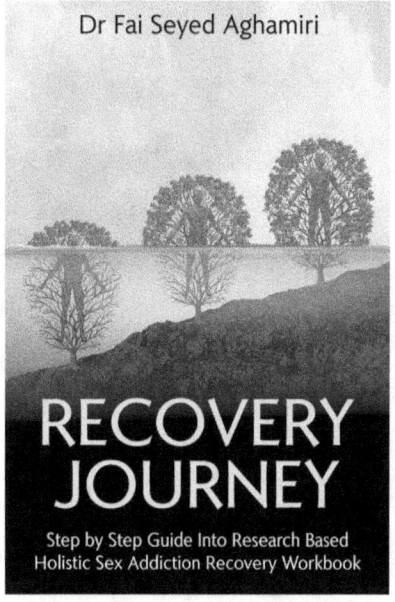